The No-Nonsense Guide to Food and Nutrition

The No-Nonsense Guide to Food and Nutrition

The Facts for Everyone . . .
by the People Who Know

MARION McGILL, M.S.
ORREA PYE, Ph.D.

Butterick Publishing

Copyright © 1978 by
Butterick Publishing
708 Third Avenue
New York, New York 10017
A Division of American Can Company

All rights reserved. No part of this book may be reproduced in any form or by any electronic or mechanical means including information storage and retrieval systems without permission in writing from the publisher (except by a reviewer who may quote brief passages in a review).

Library of Congress Cataloging in Publication Data

McGill, Marion.
   The no-nonsense guide to food and nutrition.
   Includes index.
   1. Food. 2. Nutrition. I. Pye, Orrea Florence, 1907–   joint author. II. Title.
TX353.M2517   641.1   77-92606
ISBN 0-88421-054-5

Design by Bobye G. List
Illustrations by Mel Klapholz
Manufactured in the United States of America

CONTENTS

1. A Brief History of Nutrition — 9
2. Carbohydrates and Fats — 21
3. Protein and Amino Acids — 37
4. Minerals and Water — 50
5. Vitamins — 66
6. The Recommended Dietary Allowances and the U.S. Recommended Daily Allowances for Nutrition Labeling — 94
7. Milk and Milk Products — 104
8. Protein Foods: Meat, Poultry, Fish, Eggs, and Legumes — 116
9. Fruits and Vegetables — 141
10. Foods from Grains — 158
11. Food Sources of Fat — 171

12. Convenience Foods	180
13. How to Choose a Nutritionally Balanced Diet	198
Epilogue	219
Index	221

TABLES

Alcoholic Beverages	177
The Backbone of Good Nutrition	206–207
Calories, Protein, Fat Content of Major Protein Foods	119
Proper Nutrition for Babies	217
Proper Nutrition for Children	210
Nutritive Value of Fresh Fruit as Eaten Raw	154–155
Nutritive Value of Foods from Grains as Eaten	168–169
Nutritive Value of High-Fat Foods	178–179
Nutritive Value of High Protein Foods as Eaten Cooked	122–123
Nutritive Value of Milk (Various Forms), Yogurt, Cheese	112–113
Nutritive Value of Fresh Vegetables as Eaten Cooked	156–157
Recommended Dietary Allowances	96–97
Suggested Weights for Heights	214
What We Need for Good Health (Essential Nutrients)	16–17

The No-Nonsense Guide
to Food and Nutrition

1.
A Brief History of Nutrition

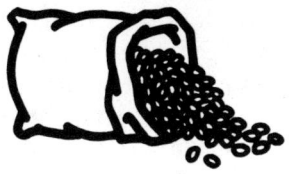

Until late in the nineteenth century, the word "nutrition" was rarely used. Food was part of our cultural heritage and experience. Each culture determined what was edible and how it was acquired, prepared, shared, and consumed. Much of this folk wisdom was sound, but many ideas about food were based on superstitions, myths, or false interpretations of observations.

There are countless examples of both accurate and inaccurate folk ideas about food. Instinctive behavior was doubtless responsible for breast feeding, but the adaptive use of milk from other animals involved reasoning more than instinct. Cooking food, perhaps initially by accident, certainly made many foods more digestible and safer for use. In time, people also learned to dry, salt, and pickle in order to save plentiful foods for later use.

From earliest times, people had to cope with many threats to their food supply. Natural disasters such as extreme heat and cold, floods, droughts, insect and fungus infestations, and earthquakes often resulted in famine. Human threats to the food supply included overpopulation, soil depletion resulting from faulty farming practices, wars, often initiated by competition for food and land, and epidemics of disease.

Fortunately, human beings proved very adaptable to different environments and sources of food. Foods that may seem unusual or even distasteful to us have been used by other people in other cultures. For example, ancient Mexicans ate grasshoppers and ants, both of which are sources of protein. Several kinds of insects were considered delicacies in Greek and Roman times, and some are still enjoyed in parts of Asia, Australia, and Africa. We can use both plant and animal foods and, within definite limits, can adjust to feast or famine. Despite this adaptability, balance in nutrition has been important throughout history.

A study of food practices of early civilizations makes it clear that humans can exist on many diverse food patterns as long as nutrient needs are met. The early Egyptians seem to have been generally well nourished on an excellent mixed diet of grains, vegetables, legumes, fruits, nuts, milk, cheese, fish, and meat, with some taboos against pork and beef. Grains, especially primitively ground wheat, predominated in the diet. Herodotus, the Greek historian of the fifth century B.C., wrote that the Egyptians were the healthiest people known, after the Libyans, who were at that time a nomadic dairying people. Surviving statues and carvings too show vigorous Egyptians.

Many early people, including those in parts of India and China, followed a vegetarian diet, making good use of legumes, along with grains. This diet is, of course, adequate if it includes a variety of complementary protein foods (see Chapter 3) and a source of vitamin B_{12}, found only in animal foods such as milk and eggs. A lacto-ovo-vegetarian (milk-and-egg) diet has always been an excellent one nutritionally. It is a diet advocated by many people today who are concerned about world hunger.

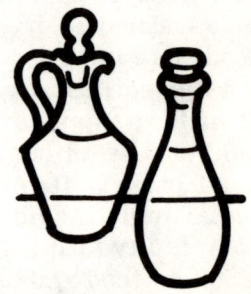

CHEMISTRY AND NUTRITION

Not until the 1600's, when an exact science of chemistry began to evolve, was the stage set for understanding physiological processes and the development of nutritional science.

The eighteenth-century French nobleman Lavoisier is called

the father of nutrition because of his understanding of how and why we breathe and the relation of breathing to energy use. Unfortunately, he died on the guillotine in 1794 at the age of 51, reportedly begging for a few weeks in which to finish his experiments.

Nineteenth-century German scientists such as Baron Justus von Liebig and Carl von Voit developed the principles of organic chemistry, with applications to energy and protein metabolism. Voit was a remarkable teacher who had two notable American students, Graham Lusk and W. O. Atwater. Atwater is often referred to as the father of American nutrition. He expanded nutrition studies in the United States after he returned from Germany, and in 1894 he persuaded Congress to provide funds to the U.S. Department of Agriculture for the first food and nutrition investigations.

In 1900 only 12 amino acids had been identified as components of dietary protein. Today we know not only that there are 22 amino acids, we also know our requirement and the function of the essential 9 discussed in Chapter 3. This advance in scientific knowledge represents the contributions of many investigators who unravelled the intricacies of protein metabolism. Even today, however, there are aspects of human need and the use of protein that are not well understood. Individual nutrition scientists differ in their recommendations for the most desirable amounts and kinds of protein foods to be consumed throughout life and in various circumstances. The Recommended Dietary Allowances (see Chapter 6) represent a composite of their opinion. Unfortunately, to add to our confusion, there are also pseudoscientists who are ill informed but who nevertheless give their views, which are sometimes conflicting and often misleading.

In the early 1900's, chemical elements present in the body were classified as they are today, as organic (carbon, hydrogen, oxygen, nitrogen) and inorganic (sulphur, phosphorus, fluorine, chlorine, iodine, silicon, sodium, potassium, calcium, magnesium, lithium, and iron). Today's inorganic list is longer, and now we also know something about the function and dietary requirement of many of these elements. Earlier, almost nothing was known about function, and nothing at all about amounts needed.

In fact, scientists did not know whether the minute amount of a mineral present in the body was there for some purpose or by contamination from the environment. It has taken 75 years of intense scientific effort to puzzle out what we know about minerals today (Chapter 4), and there are still many gaps in our understanding, such as the interrelationships among the minerals and other nutrients.

"Protective" Foods

At the turn of the century, Atwater was working with a nutrition staff at the U.S. Department of Agriculture. He began not only to analyze foods chemically but to survey the diets of people in different areas of the United States to see what foods were "protective" in keeping families healthy. Protective foods include foods in their natural state, such as milk, eggs, vegetables, fruits, and whole grains. Food guides were worked out to help families with food selection. The emphasis was on protein foods and on those containing carbohydrates and fats for energy. Because little was understood about the need for amino acids and minerals, and nothing at all about vitamins, the advice given about the choice of foods was not always the best in terms of today's greater knowledge. For example, much more protein than needed was advised, setting a pattern for a diet high in animal foods and low in fruits and vegetables. Some people still eat more meat than needed and count calories without reference to other vitally important nutrients.

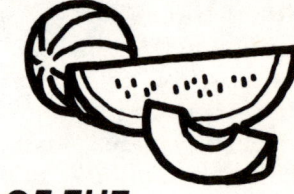

VITAMINS: DISCOVERIES OF THE TWENTIETH CENTURY

Nothing was known about vitamins until about 1906, when an English scientist, Frederick Hopkins, found that it was necessary to add a small amount of milk to the purified laboratory ration of rats in order for them to survive and grow. He theorized that the lack of certain unknown factors in foods might be the causes of many diseases such as rickets and scurvy. Prior to 1906, it had been recognized that certain human diseases were cured or prevented by certain foods. British sailors, for example, were called limeys because their shipboard provisions included limes or lemons to ward off the dread scurvy, caused by vitamin C deficiency.

Some observers noted that the widespread disease beriberi developed in peoples who ate polished rice but not in those who ate unpolished rice. Rice polishings or bran were therefore used as a cure for beriberi. But what was it in the rice bran that was effective? In 1912 a Polish chemist, Casimir Funk, suggested the name "beriberi vitamine" for a substance he had isolated from rice bran. The term *vitamin(e)* came to be used for all the mysterious substances needed in very small amount which were not the previously recognized nutritional substances—that is carbohydrates, fats, proteins, and minerals.

NUTRITION PIONEERS

The twentieth century has been an era of tremendous research activity into the riddles of nutrition. There have been many noteworthy nutrition investigators and teachers, far too many to list other than a few pioneers.

Lafayette Mendel and coworkers at Yale University made key advances in our knowledge of protein, amino acids, and other nutrients. They were inspiring teachers of the new nutrition science and produced a long line of successors working throughout the United States.

Elmer McCollum, who worked first at the University of Wisconsin and later at John Hopkins University, was an outstanding leader. He wrote about his early experiments in trying to rear rats on purified rations and, like Hopkins, found it impossible without some milk. Adding fat to his ration, McCollum found butterfat effective, but not lard or olive oil. After many trials he and coworkers identified fat-soluble "A," later called vitamin A, in 1914.

Henry Sherman and coworkers at Columbia University were outstanding investigators as well as teachers, beginning in the early 1900's. Sherman, a prolific writer, suggested human requirements for protein, calcium, phosphorus, and other nutrients which are close to those on which the Recommended Dietary Allowances are based.

W. C. Rose, a student of Mendel's who went to the University of Illinois, established basic requirements for the essential amino acids, using volunteer college students as subjects.

Mary Swartz Rose of Teachers College, Columbia University, was a student of Mendel's (1907–1909) and a student and colleague of Sherman's. Her noteworthy research focused on practical dietary concerns. Her teaching and development of training programs for dietitians and nutritionists were outstanding, as were her many books and articles directed to college students, teachers, nurses, and general readers.

In the following decades Agnes Fay Morgan of the University of California at Berkeley (1915 to 1954) was an outstanding nutrition scientist, researcher, and teacher. She had wide interests in research in applied nutrition and was the author of many publications.

Lydia Roberts, a contemporary at the University of Chicago, was another renowned teacher and eminent contributor to research in applied nutrition. Her book, *Nutrition Work with Children*, published in 1927, is a classic in its field.

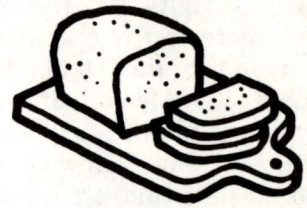

WAR AND NUTRITION

It is ironic that it was during two world wars that people in the United States became more aware of nutrition. This awareness led to progress in improving our dietary habits and also stimulated the government to take constructive action. By World War I, nutrition knowledge was sufficiently advanced so that dietary advice could be directed at the population under food rationing. Food conservation and the use of less meat and more vegetables were emphasized.

During World War II, President Franklin Roosevelt held a National Nutrition Conference for Defense. In addition, the Food and Nutrition Board of the National Research Council was formed as part of the National Academy of Science. Enrichment programs were initiated, taking advantage of new food technology and the availability of chemically isolated vitamins. As time has gone on, enrichment has led to fortification practices at high levels and including other nutrients not always present in the natural food (see Chapter 10).

FORTIFICATION

A question about current fortification of foods that has not been thoroughly answered is how well the pure chemical nutrients used in fortification are absorbed by our digestive tracts under different conditions. In general, it seems that the body uses these purified vitamins and minerals very well. However, we also know that the essential nutrients must all be present in the right balance and available in the body for our best health.

Many foods and food products have nutrients added to bring them up to the level of the U.S. Recommended Daily Allowances used in labeling (see Chapter 6). Some nutritionists are concerned about the addition to highly processed foods of relatively few nutrients in fairly large amounts. Certain questions arise from this practice. Traditional foods are the naturally occurring foods. (We are avoiding the term *natural foods* because we believe it has been used indiscriminately in advertising and by the health food industry.) Since some of the trace or minor nutrients present in traditional foods (earlier called "protective" foods) are not restored to processed foods, could nutritional imbalance occur in cases where convenience foods are used almost exclusively? At present we do not know enough about the requirements of trace nutrients to make a truly balanced synthetic food for humans.

HEALTH AND MODERN NUTRITION

It is not really possible to say on the basis of a few weeks or months that such and such a diet is nutritionally satisfactory. For example, body stores may mask a diet's inadequacy on a short-term basis. Time is a vital factor, as changes in body cells can occur slowly and not be detected for years.

Food technology has been a great asset over the years and can continue to be if sensibly used. It helps to preserve foods and make them available throughout the year. But some food engineering, particularly of convenience products, may well be ahead of our nutritional knowledge.

Marketing techniques and intensive food advertising in all media hard sell these new products. There are differences of opinion about these tactics, but certainly all the additives developed to enhance color, taste, texture, and shelf life make it hard for governmental consumer protection agencies to keep up with evaluating the safety of these new products.

Today a consumer needs greater nutritional knowledge than ever to select an adequate, well-balanced diet for all family members.

About 50 nutrients are known to be essential for proper growth and good health from infancy to old age. As this new science of nutrition progresses and additional research is done, other nutrients and their interrelationships may be discovered and a greater knowledge of those presently known will come about.

WHAT WE NEED FOR GOOD HEALTH

Water	Transporter of nutrients	
Three sources of energy	Carbohydrates, fats, and proteins	
Eight essential amino acids	Components, not synthesized by our bodies, and needed for building and maintaining body protein	
	Isoleucine	Phenylalanine
	Leucine	Threonine
	Lysine	Tryptophan
	Methionine	Valine
Ninth amino acid in childhood	Histidine	
Nonessential amino acids	Additional nitrogen	
Twenty-one minerals: for making bones and teeth, maintaining the chemical balance of our body fluids, and initiating metabolic actions	*Macrominerals*	
	Calcium	Sodium
	Phosphorus	Potassium
	Magnesium	Chloride
	Sulphur	
	Trace minerals	
	Iodine	Molybdenum
	Iron	Selenium
	Copper	Chromium
	Cobalt	Nickel
	Manganese	Tin
	Zinc	Vanadium
	Fluorine	Silicon

Fourteen vitamins: to work with amino acids and minerals in all body functions	*Four fat-soluble vitamins*
	Vitamin A Vitamin E
	Vitamin D Vitamin K
	Ten water-soluble vitamins
	Thiamin Vitamin B_{12}
	Riboflavin Pantothenic
	Niacin acid
	Vitamin B_6 Biotin
	Folacin Choline
	     Ascorbic Acid
	     (vitamin C)

One essential fatty acid: for growth in infancy and healthy skin	Linoleic acid
Fiber: for proper functioning and healthy digestive tract	Indigestible carbohydrates (cellulose and pectin) from whole grains, vegetables, and fruits
Possibly unknown nutrients	

The Dangers of Feasting

We mentioned earlier that within definite limits people can adjust to either feast or famine. There are grave dangers at either extreme. Over the last few decades, affluent America has had almost too much good food to eat. Dr. Mark Hegsted, a leading nutrition biochemist at Harvard, stated recently that in the past the first concern of U.S. nutritionists was the prevention of nutritional deficiency. To assure an adequate intake of essential nutrients for everyone is still a fundamental and vital goal. There is still undernutrition in the U.S.A. But today, many major health problems are associated with "overnutrition"—excessive consumption of food. Thirty or forty years ago people suffered from pellagra, rickets, and other illnesses caused by nutritional deficiency. Nutritional advice at that time was, in essence, "eat more of everything." Dr. Hegsted points out that large segments of the food industry will not be happy with the guidance to limit some of the food we eat, which is the advice we need to stress today, but this new emphasis is in our best interests.

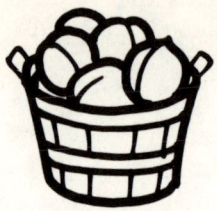

Keys to Good Health

People must now be more discriminating and eat enough of the foods needed for good health, but they must also avoid gaining too much weight. Specifically, they must limit those foods associated with certain kinds of heart disease, hypertension, cancer, diabetes, and other degenerative diseases which constitute major health problems in America today. These conditions are under active research, and we are learning more about their prevention and cure. Although we do not have all the answers, by any means, in terms of diet or other factors, certain guidelines do exist. For example, too many high-calorie foods should be avoided. High-fat diets are definitely suspect (see Chapters 3 and 12) and high meat consumption, also associated with saturated fat, is suggested as related to cancer of the colon. High sugar consumption and obesity are suspect as causes of diabetes. The importance of low-salt diets in treatment of hypertension seems to be established. It is less clear whether table salt (sodium chloride) is a cause of hypertension, but it certainly seems desirable not to use salt or other sodium compounds to excess. Many chemical additives used in convenience foods are sodium compounds, and one wonders whether this fact is taken into account sufficiently by manufacturers and consumers.

In general, Americans seem to believe that if a little is good, more is better. This is definitely not true in nutrition, as statements in the current publication of the Recommended Dietary Allowances point out. "We are aware of no convincing evidence of unique health benefits occurring from consumption of a large excess of any one nutrient," and "Claims that large intakes of individual nutrients will cure non-nutritional diseases should be viewed with skepticism since they can encourage delay in the diagnosis and treatment of diseases and symptoms that should have prompt and appropriate medical attention" are examples of such warnings.

FOOD, ENERGY, AND THE FUTURE

There are reasons other than health why high intakes of calories and animal protein are not desirable. One such reason is the world food economy. Cattle and other cud-chewing animals that graze on range land and digest fibrous materials inedible for humans have a definite place in balanced land and food management. But in recent years Americans have come to demand more (and more tender) beef, produced by fattening cattle on grain in feed lots. This feeding practice not only adds more saturated fat to the meat but is very uneconomical. We lose energy and protein in converting plant protein to meat protein. Economists warn that a rich minority cannot continue to pull the price of grain out of the reach of poor people. We can eat "lower on the food chain" by using more vegetables and cereals for direct protein and less of the indirect animal protein. The use of milk and eggs as protein sources is less wasteful of protein and energy not only because the conversion factor is less but also because no animal is killed or eliminated as a food producer.

Americans not only tend to eat too much, but we are wasteful with food, as with other natural resources. A recent study of food waste by anthropologists in Tucson, Arizona, indicated that in 1974 Tucson families wasted about 9½ tons of edible food. It was also estimated that enough meat, poultry, or fish was discarded in a week to supply the protein needs of 4,000 people over the same period of time.

In 1977, we had a plentiful supply of grain in the United States. In fact, farmers were subsidized not to plant wheat. But drought and other unfavorable climatic conditions can change crop success to failure very quickly. Moreover, while fewer births are holding the population down, longer life for many, plus immigration, means our total population is still increasing. Thus, we will continue to need more food to feed people in the United States.

Many thoughtful people are concerned about our energy-intensive food system today. Through agribusiness and its extensive use of fertilizers, irrigation, pesticides, and machines, we have increased crop yields per acre. We have also lost much prime farmland and many small family farms by paving them over for suburban developments.

Food, land, water, and energy are closely linked. As far as

food is concerned, there are multiple reasons for conservation—improved nutrition and health, economy, population pressures, and international concerns. We learn from history that humans can adapt to change. We also note that when past civilizations failed to adapt appropriately, they fell.

Food conservation is really not difficult to practice. The major points are:

- Eat less meat protein and fat and more vegetable protein.
- Use more naturally occuring foods and fewer convenience foods, which take energy to make.
- Waste less food.

We can teach our children more frugal eating habits.

What we save by food conservation can begin to help to ease the energy shortage. And in the long run, our children will be better nourished, healthier, and more able to cope with problems of possible food shortages in the future.

2.
Carbohydrates and Fats

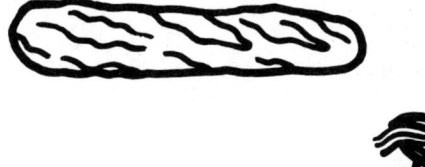

FOOD ENERGY

To live we must have three things—oxygen, water, and food. We breathe oxygen from the air, we get water from nature's supply, and we grow plants and raise animals for food. Our first need from food is energy, for all the functions of our bodies and everything we do; to grow from an infant into an adult; and to maintain our adult bodies in good health.

After the discovery was made that we also require protein, for maintenance and repair of the body, foods were classified on the basis of the then known substances that they contain in the greatest amount—that is, carbohydrate, protein, and fat. But today we know that no one food is a source of just one nutrient and that we must think of foods according to their complete nutritional value.

The major source of energy should be the carbohydrate foods. They are the most economical in terms of purchase price and agricultural resources and the most completely utilized in energy metabolism. Food fats, the most concentrated sources of energy, have become the major source of calories in the American diet today. Protein foods can be sources of energy as well as of protein-building material. Fats and proteins used for energy are covered later in this chapter and in the following one.

Energy and Calories

Just as a lump of sugar can be burned to give off heat, a form of energy, so blood sugar burns in the tissue cells to give energy regulated by a series of reactions that keeps our body heat constant. This heat can be measured in calories. A calorie is the amount of heat required to raise 1 cubic centimeter of water from 15 to 16 degrees centigrade. In the science of nutrition, the measure of the potential energy of a food is given in kilocalories, which is 1,000 calories. A kilocalorie is sometimes written as *Calorie* with a capital *C*, or abbreviated to *KCal*. The caloric value of fat averages 9 kilocalories per gram. Nature has the amazing ability to compact more than twice as much energy or twice as many calories into fat as in an equal weight of carbohydrate. The caloric value of carbohydrate and protein used in the body for energy averages 4 kilocalories per gram.

CARBOHYDRATE FOODS

Some carbohydrate foods, especially those that have the carbohydrate in a complex form such as starch, have been downgraded in the American diet. But these starches are a better source of energy for athletes, laborers, and growing children than are fats and proteins. Recent research is showing that these more complex forms that take longer to digest and process in the body, usually accompanied by indigestible carbohydrate or fiber which helps to maintain normal digestion and absorption, are better for all of us than simple or refined sugars. It is true that a large segment of the population do little physical work and have a low expenditure of energy, so the amount of food they can consume in addition to the foods that provide essential nutrients is limited. But to reduce the intake of carbohydrate foods to extremely low levels to accomplish this energy balance is dangerous.

Naturally occurring foods generally considered high in carbohydrate include the cereal grains; vegetables that are 15 percent or more carbohydrate, including the legumes, and fruits that are 15 percent or more carbohydrate. However, all fruits and vegetables are carbohydrate foods. All of the above make valuable contributions to our vitamin and mineral needs, and the cereal grains, legumes, and some vegetables make valuable contributions to the protein or amino acid pool of our bodies as well. Thus the carbohydrate foods should be judged by their overall nutritive value as well as our best sources of energy.

Carbohydrates are sugars, starches, pectins, and cellulose (fiber) made by plants and milk sugar, and glycogen made by animals.

All living matter is made of carbon atoms linked to each other and linked with a variety of other elements. This gives varieties of living matter their distinct identities. The links that hold the atoms together are called bonds, and each atom has a specific number of bonds that determines how it can unite with other atoms. The carbon atom has four, oxygen has two, hydrogen has one, and nitrogen has three. These are the principal basic elements of carbohydrate. In the simplest form, the carbon atoms are linked to one another in short chains that make up a molecule. From a few to hundreds of molecules are linked together to form compounds. The sugar of your blood, glucose, is a molecule 6 carbons long. The starch of potatoes is a compound made of hundreds of glucose molecules linked together.

How We Use the Food Made by Plants

A growing plant has mechanisms for taking carbon dioxide (carbon and oxygen) from the air, hydrogen from the water, and nitrogen from the soil to grow into a mature plant that will blossom and produce a fruit or seed.

The plant links up these elements by an exceedingly complex interaction of enzymes, the green pigment chlorophyll, the energy from the sun. Some of the enzymes that are formed contain the vitamins we need and play a role again in the release of this energy in our body cells.

$$\text{6 carbon dioxide} + \text{6 Water} \xrightarrow[\text{chlorophyll}]{\text{sunlight}} \text{glucose (sugar)} + \text{6 oxygen}$$
$$CO_2 + H_2O \xrightarrow[\text{chlorophyll}]{\text{sunlight}} C_6H_{12}O_6 + O_2$$

Animals and humans use plants for food by an even more complicated series of reactions. First, the food eaten is changed by digestive enzymes, which unhook some of the linkages between the carbon atoms to reduce the food compounds to molecules again. In this form they pass into the cells of the intestinal wall. On the other side of the wall, the linkages are unhooked even further, again by the action of enzymes and also by hormones, and then rebuilt into new molecules which you require for energy and repair. If you are under 25 years, you also use energy for growth. (Women have increased energy needs during pregnancy and when they breast-feed their babies.)

The human body is really a remarkable chemistry system. We eat animal and plant foods, which are distinctive chemical compounds, and our system transforms those foods into the basic molecules from which they were made. Some of the molecules are unhooked even further into atoms with the release of energy. And some of the molecules are linked in new ways to build the distinctive compounds of which we are made.

The Chemistry of Carbohydrates

All carbohydrates are made of three elements—carbon, hydrogen, and oxygen. An infinite number of atoms of these are arranged in an infinite number of ways to build all the carbohydrate material in nature. The simplest of these are monosaccharides, or sugars. Trioses are sugars that are 3 linked carbons; tetroses are 4 linked carbons; pentoses are 5 linked carbons. But it is a 6-carbon, or hexose, form, commonly called glucose, that is the most important carbohydrate substance in human metabolism. It has 6 carbon atoms linked together holding 12 hydrogen atoms and 6 oxygen atoms with its other bonds. It is written $C_6H_{12}O_6$.

$$\begin{array}{c} C \!\!\stackrel{\displaystyle H}{=}\!\! O \\ | \\ H-C-OH \\ | \\ HO-C-H \\ | \\ H-C-OH \\ | \\ H-C-OH \\ | \\ {}^{H}\!\!\diagdown\!\!{}_{}\!\!\!C-OH \\ {}^{H}\!\!\diagup \end{array}$$

Changing the order of the Hs and OHs results in slightly different hexoses. The most important rearranged forms in human nutrition are fructose and galactose.

Glucose occurs in the free state in ripe fruit, flowers, leaves, roots, and sap of plants; in the body, it is the sugar in the blood.
Fructose is found in ripe fruit, honey, molasses, and syrups.
Galactose is not found free; it is linked with a glucose molecule in lactose, the sugar of milk.

When two monosaccharides are linked as in lactose they are called disaccharides. Familiar disaccharides are:

Maltose is sugar formed in malting grain—one glucose linked to another.
Sucrose is a glucose linked to a fructose, found naturally in ripe fruit and commercially refined from sugar beets and sugar cane to become all the forms of table sugar.

When more than ten monosaccharides are linked, they form the poly-saccharides, which are the starches, pectins, and cellulose of plants. Animals and man link glucose units to make glycogen. But no matter which form carbohydrate is in when it is eaten, all digestible sugars and starches are changed during the process of digestion into the one simple form—glucose. Pectins and cellulose are indigestible carbohydrates referred to as fiber.

Glucose into Energy

Just as the process of digestion is a complex and almost miraculous series of chemical reactions whereby the food we eat is reduced to a form in which it can pass through the cells of the intestinal wall, the chain of reactions in which the food is used by the body is even more miraculous and complex. This is the process of metabolism. And just as we understand many of the digestive processes—that an enzyme in saliva starts the digestion of carbohydrates, that hydrochloric acid and enzymes in the stomach digest protein—we now understand many of the reactions of metabolism and can even write them as chemical equations. You needn't know all these in order to understand nutrition, but it is important to have some concept of energy metabolism because all the food sources of energy, the proteins and fats as well as the carbohydrates, end up going through the same energy-releasing cycle. It is just before this cycle that the energy-giving units are made ready to be used as immediate energy or are converted to stored energy, or body fat.

When the whole complex system of exchanges in which energy is released go on in your body cells, carbon dioxide and water are produced. The carbon dioxide is carried in your blood stream to the lungs and exhaled, the water carried to your kidneys and excreted.

Energy Need is Constant

The body's need for basic energy for living processes is constant. Even at times of complete rest the muscles of the heart and lungs are working, the temperature of the body is maintained, and metabolic processes are going on. In the tissue cells the release of energy for these functions goes on continuously. Yet there does not have to be a steady stream of energy-giving nutrients entering the blood stream from the digestive system. People can go for quite long periods without food because the body has a very efficient storage system for energy nutrients. There is no need to eat constantly. This storage system served people much better in the past, and serves better where food is scarce today as compared with societies where food is abundant; for it is through this storage system that all energy supplies in excess of the body needs are stored as extra weight.

In the normal chain of events glucose passes through the intestinal wall into the bloodstream. Yet no matter how much food is consumed, the glucose level of the blood is remarkably constant. In the normal person it does rise immediately after a meal, but it drops to a constant level again in one to two hours. The blood carries the glucose molecules to the liver and the muscles, and those not immediately needed are linked together again (the reverse of the unlinking by the digestive enzymes) into glycogen. The glycogen in the muscles remains there until it is used by the muscles. When energy is needed, the glycogen is changed back to glucose and then through all the subsequent reactions to release that energy.

The glycogen in the liver is more continually drawn on since one of the important functions of the liver is to keep the blood glucose at a constant level. After a meal, the blood loaded with glucose from the digestive tract goes to the liver, where the excess glucose is removed and changed to glycogen. The blood circulates through the body constantly, giving up its glucose to the cells for countless uses; it then returns to the liver for another supply. The liver alternates the processes of changing glucose from food to glycogen (for storage) to blood glucose (for use as energy).

The amount of glycogen that can be stored is limited. Muscles can take from 200 to 250 grams and the liver about 100 grams. But when those storage depots are filled, the glucose level of the blood must still not be allowed to rise, so the other storage system for energy comes into action, the conversion to fat.

Recommended Dietary Allowance (RDA)

Carbohydrate foods are readily available and inexpensive. They have traditionally been a mainstay in meal patterns, but with the promotion of the undesirable low-carbohydrate regimes prescribed as a means of losing excess weight, a deficiency of carbohydrate is possible.

The eighth edition (1974) of the Food and Nutrition Board's Recommended Dietary Allowances states that it is desirable to include some carbohydrate in the diet to avoid ketosis; excessive breakdown of body protein; loss of minerals, especially sodium; and involuntary dehydration. From 50 to 100 grams of digestible carbohydrate a day will offset the undesirable metabolic responses resulting from high-fat diets and fasting.

Indigestible Carbohydrate: Fiber

The most complex carbohydrates are the pectins and celluloses. These substances are made of hundreds of linked molecules and provide the structure of plants (stems, leaves, fruits). They are digested by ruminant animals but are mostly unchanged in the human digestive system. The celluloses, in particular, add bulk to the digestive residue, and there is increasing evidence that the health of especially the lower digestive tract is benefited by including a certain amount of fiber in the diet. There is also some evidence that fiber may trap and prevent the absorption of some of the cholesterol present in the digesting food.

FATS

Fats are made of the same three elements as carbohydrates—carbon, hydrogen, and oxygen. The way they are put together is similar but the proportion of each is different. Fats are made with less oxygen and have two major units. One unit is 3 linked-up carbon atoms, each also linked to hydrogen and oxygen molecules to make a substance called glycerol in biochemistry and glycerine in the drugstore.

The other unit is 3 even-numbered chains of carbons which vary in length from 2 to 20. These chains also contain hydrogen and are called fatty acids. In a fat, each of the 3 carbons of glycerol is attached to a fatty acid, and the substance formed is called a triglyceride. In some fatty acids each carbon atom, in addition to being linked in a chain to 2 other carbons, is linked on each side to hydrogen. Each carbon can make only 4 links, and such a fatty acid is termed *saturated* because all the links are used.

$$-\overset{H}{\underset{H}{C}}-\overset{H}{\underset{H}{C}}-\overset{H}{\underset{H}{C}}-\overset{H}{\underset{H}{C}}\rightarrow$$

In other fatty acids, a pair of carbons may be linked in a chain to other carbons, but to hydrogen only on one side. This leaves 2 links free—which they hold between them as a double bond—and the fatty acid is termed *unsaturated*.

$$-\overset{H}{\underset{H}{C}}-\overset{H}{C}=\overset{H}{C}-\overset{H}{\underset{H}{C}}\rightarrow$$

When a fatty acid has only one pair of carbons with a double bond, it is called monounsaturated. When it has more than one pair, it is called *polyunsaturated*.

glycerol

C — $-\overset{H}{\underset{H}{C}}-\overset{H}{\underset{H}{C}}-\overset{H}{\underset{H}{C}}-\overset{H}{\underset{H}{C}}\rightarrow$ saturated fatty acid

C — $-\overset{H}{\underset{H}{C}}-\overset{H}{C}=\overset{H}{C}-\overset{H}{\underset{H}{C}}\rightarrow$ mono-unsaturated fatty acid

C — $-\overset{H}{\underset{H}{C}}-\overset{H}{C}=\overset{H}{C}-\overset{H}{\underset{H}{C}}-\overset{H}{\underset{H}{C}}-\overset{H}{C}=\overset{H}{C}-\overset{H}{\underset{}{C}}\rightarrow$ poly-unsaturated fatty acid

A triglyceride

A diglyceride is a glycerol connected to only two fatty acids, and a monoglyceride is attached to only one fatty acid. These are formed when fat is digested, and they act to emulsify other fat in the digestive process. They can also be made from fat. Both of these substances may appear in the ingredient listings of food products as emulsifiers.

Fatty Acids

There are a great number of fatty acids. They differ in the length of their carbon chains and their degree of saturation. Both these factors affect the characteristics of the fats in which they are combined. The fatty acids most commonly found in food fats are listed below. In ingredient listings on food packages, words like stearate, palmitate, and others are just food fats by their technical name. The simplest fatty acid is acetic acid with 2 carbon atoms (the acid of vinegar).

Saturated Fatty Acid	*Number of Carbon Atoms*
Acetic	2
Butyric (gives butter its flavor)	4
Caproic	6
Caprylic	8
Capric	10
Lauric	12
Myristic	14
Palmitic	16
Stearic	18

Unsaturated Fatty Acid	*Number of Carbon Atoms*
Palmitoleic	16
Oleic	18
Linoleic	18
Linolenic	18
Arachidonic	20

All fats as they occur naturally in foods are made of a mixture of saturated and unsaturated fatty acids. They are also made of mixtures of short- and long-chain fatty acids. No natural fat is made of glycerol and only saturated fatty acids, or of only unsaturated fatty acids. The same is true of our own body fat if we follow a conventional diet. The only fat in our diet that contains a glycerol combined with three saturated fatty acids is solid processed fat or shortening that has had hydrogen added—thus called hydrogenated vegetable oil or shortening.

The short-chain fatty acids, up to 12 carbons, are liquid at room temperature. Butter becomes soft at room temperature because it contains short-chain fatty acids. But long-chain fatty acids that are unsaturated are also liquid at room temperature. The vegetable fats like corn oil and soybean oil, which are high in oleic and linoleic acids are examples. Coconut oil has a high proportion of saturated fatty acid and is an exception to the generality that animal fats are saturated fats and vegetable oils are unsaturated.

Fats that are made mostly of saturated fatty acids are more stable than those made of a high proportion of unsaturated ones. Oxygen can link with the double bonds and cause the fat to change or become rancid. For this reason, in the ingredient listing of convenience foods that contain fats or were processed in fat (like potato chips), you will find additives called antioxidants. Vitamin E is an antioxidant that is present naturally in oils and fats. It is also added to food products to prevent changes or oxidation of the fat. Rancid fats, in addition to having an unpleasant taste, may be harmful.

Energy Storage

The need for energy is constant for living processes and increases as your activity does. But you do not have to be continually taking in or eating a constant source of energy because your body is able to store energy.

The energy from all the foods you eat is stored in two forms, glycogen and fat. Here is what happens. All the carbohydrate foods are digested to glucose which can then pass through the intestinal wall into the blood stream. The glucose is taken to the liver, and in a matter of hours some of it is linked into glycogen. Glycogen is our body's form of complex carbohydrate and our form of quickly available stored energy. When the glycogen stores are filled, the remaining glucose is changed into fat and stored in our fat cells to be a later supply of constant energy.

In a similar manner, the energy from extra protein is stored as fat. The protein foods you eat are digested to amino acids so they can pass from the intestine into the blood stream. Like glucose, they go to the liver for a sort of processing before they are circulated in the general blood stream. In a matter of hours, they are used by the body cells to synthesize new protein to replace old or worn out cells. Any amino acids left in the blood stream after the immediate body needs for protein synthesis are satisfied are changed into two chemical units. The unit that made them amino acids is discarded; the other unit is changed to fat and stored for its energy.

The fat foods you eat in a meal are also digested into their components, but not quite so completely. They pass through the intestinal wall, partly as fatty acids and glycerol and partly as emulsified mono- and diglycerides and fats (triglycerides). Then they follow one of two routes. The glycerol and fatty acids go via the blood stream to the liver, and the others go through the lymph system and then to the liver.

The liver is the center of fat metabolism. In a relatively short space of time it is able to convert the fat components from digestion into forms used immediately by the body or into the form for storage. In order to do this, the liver requires choline and vitamin B_{12} among other substances, to prevent the fat from accumulating within it.

The fats that the liver makes from the supply of glucose and from extra amino acids follow a pattern of a genetic code; they contain both saturated and unsaturated fatty acids. The synthesis is controlled by hormones, and each step requires enzymes that contain vitamins or trace minerals. The process is a very efficient one of energy storage. When converted to fat, the carbohydrate and protein you have eaten are changed so that the fat you store has more than twice the energy per gram than the original substances.

The fats that are formed from food fats may be different. Some food fat can be stored without any rearranging of the fatty-acid units so that the composition of the food fats can somewhat affect the composition of your body fat. However, you should not think of food fats in terms of which is best for storage, but in terms of which is best for health. Keep to a low intake of fat foods and don't let fat storage build up to overweight.

Fats do not circulate in the blood as fats, but are linked up with protein, phosphorus, and other substances, including cholesterol. Some of these compounds have other purposes as well as transporting fat to storage cells. In the storage cell, the fat is mainly in the form of a triglyceride along with the enzymes necessary to make it quickly convertible to energy.

The concept that fat tissue is inert and unchanging is far from true. It is very active and constantly changing. When no energy is being supplied by digestion, the fats (triglycerides) in storage are picked up and transported to cells where energy is required. At one time it was thought that triglycerides had to be turned into glucose before they could be used, but recent research has shown that muscles and vital organs can use fatty acids directly. Only the brain and nervous system cannot do this and require the liver to convert the fatty acids to glucose for their energy needs.

The process of turning fats into energy is a long, complicated series of repeating chemical reactions as each pair of carbons is split off and ends up as carbon dioxide and water, with the release of energy. The body cells do this at an incredible speed, and the process requires enzymes, which require vitamins and minerals in their own makeup.

The main concept to grasp with regard to food and energy supplies is balance. During a meal and from four to six hours after, energy is being used directly or being put into storage. In the hours following, the storage is used. If you constantly put more into storage than you use up, you will gain weight in the form of fat. "Everything I eat turns to fat" is a saying that has a great degree of truth in it. Everything you eat in excess of your needs for energy and replacement of protein cells is actually turned into fat. There is no limit to the amount of fat the body can store.

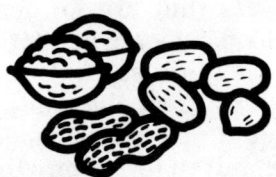

Fat and Cholesterol

The role of cholesterol in our bodies, the amount of it in our food, and the part it plays in our health have undergone much study and are still being studied and assessed.

Cholesterol is a vital substance of your brain and nervous system. It is present in your organs, more in some than others, and is found in almost all tissue cells. In your skin, in one of its forms, it is a source of vitamin D on exposure to the sun. It is needed in the synthesis of some hormones. It is used in digestion, especially of fats, when it is converted by the liver into bile acids.

About 2 grams of cholesterol are made in your body each day. Usually your body keeps a balance between the cholesterol you get from foods and the amount synthesized. When you eat more food cholesterol, more cholesterol products are eliminated by way of your digestive tract. Fiber and other dietary factors play a role in the amount absorbed or discarded.

Some cholesterol circulates in your blood and can be measured in a blood sample. In a healthy person the level in the blood is usually quite constant, though it goes up a bit as you get older. In some types of heart disease the level is elevated. For this reason doctors use the level of cholesterol in the blood as a means of diagnosing these conditions.

The Need for Fat

Since fat seems to be one of the factors in some types of heart disease you may well wonder if you will be better off not eating any. But you do require a certain amount of fat both in your food and on your body. Here are the reasons:

- There is one fatty acid we must get from food—linoleic acid.
- The fats in your food carry with them the fat-soluble vitamins—A, D, E, and K.
- Fats prolong the digestion time of a meal so that you are more satisfied and you get hungry less quickly.
- Fats make foods more flavorful; many flavors such as the oils in spices, blend with the fats.
- Fats are the most concentrated food source of energy. Fats, like carbohydrates, "spare" protein. When present as a source of food energy, fats allow proteins to be used for their more important functions instead of being used up for their energy.
- Some stores of fat in your body are around your internal organs, acting as protection or cushioning against shock or injury, especially the kidneys.
- Some of the fat is under your skin, and there it acts as an insulation against cold and helps keep your internal temperature constant.

Two Essential Fatty Acids

Linoleic acid is the only fatty acid you do not synthesize, and you must get it from food. Arachidonic acid, which you also need, can be made from linoleic acid if it is not supplied by food. Linoleic acid is not likely to be lacking in a well-rounded adult diet since the adult requirement is low. But because it is essential for growth, it is important in the food of children. In cases where there is a constant lack, the child will develop a skin condition similar to eczema.

There has been a recommended allowance suggested for these fatty acids in relation to the calories in the diet. In the food intake of infants and children, 3 percent of the total calories should be from linoleic acid; in the adult diet, 2 percent of the calories is sufficient. Unsaturated fats from both animal and vegetable sources contain linoleic acid, but the vegetable sources are best.

How Much Fat Should We Eat?

For most nutrients there is an RDA based on minimum amounts. In the case of fat it would seem we must set a maximum recommended amount. With our high standard of living and the abundant quantity and choice of foods, we seem to be developing a new set of nutritional diseases. These are not deficiency diseases, but ones of overeating, or malnutrition in the sense of too much fat both eaten and stored. Three fat-related diseases are of much concern today: obesity or excess weight in the form of fat; cancer of the breast and of the colon; and atherosclerosis and coronary heart disease. Atherosclerosis is the formation of a fatty plaque on the walls of the arteries, making the artery smaller in diameter. Coronary heart disease develops when this occurs in the major arteries of the heart. It causes a decrease in blood supply, and a consequent decrease in oxygen and energy for the heart muscle.

Three recommendations can be made to help in the control of these diseases.

- Decrease your fat intake. It is generally thought that 35 percent of the calories you need each day and no more should come from fat. This is fat that you see as oil in an oil and vinegar salad dressing and fat you do not see in cake mixes and the glossy coating on snack food. If you need 1800 calories a day then you should have no more than 630 calories as fat, which comes to 70 grams. Of the 70 grams of fat in a usual food intake, 35 grams is usually unseen in meat, cheese, pastries, and so forth. As visible fat, the other 35 grams is about 1½ tablespoons of butter or margarine and 1 tablespoon of salad oil.
- Balance the fats in your foods between unsaturated and saturated fats (in general from both animal and vegetable sources). Continuing research indicates that an intake of fats from mostly polyunsaturated fatty acids is not desirable.

✔ People with some heart conditions should choose foods that are low in fats of the saturated fatty-acid type and that are low in cholesterol. The chief food factors in heart disease seem to be the level of fat, especially saturated fat, in the diet and the level of fat storage—that is, the amount a person is overweight. (There are nonfood risk factors as well, of course, which don't concern us here.)

Despite the publicity these fat-related diseases have been given, there has been a steady rise in our consumption of fat even in the last decade. And surprising as it may seem, this increase has been in our intake of cooking fats and salad oils. Vegetable oils are used in many "convenience" products like frozen French-fried foods. These are a lot of trouble to make at home so people ate less of them before they became widely available in packaged form. The consumption of commercially prepared French-fried potatoes last year was over 1.5 billion pounds. Advertising and articles on fat and health often give a false sense of security in suggesting that unsaturated fats, especially polyunsaturated fats, are less likely to create health problems. The recommendation that polyunsaturated fats be increased in the diet does not mean in addition to other fat but in proportion to other fat.

FAT CONSUMPTION

Year	Total Fat Per Day	Vegetable Fat	Polyunsaturated Fat	Saturated Fat
1913	125gm	17%	11%	50%
1963	145gm	30%	30%	
1973	155gm	40%	24%	55%

Some say that happiness is never having to say you're on a diet. Obesity is primarily caused by a constant intake of more food energy than is used up—simply, eating too much for one's activity. Fats are the most concentrated source of energy, and our intake of fat has been steadily rising. So it would seem that a lot of our extra food energy is coming from fat.

A diet plan for losing weight that is balanced for all nutrients with restricted calories or energy is presented in chapter 13. If your weight is normal, you have less likelihood of developing either fat-related heart diseases or cancer. If you have these conditions, they are beyond the scope of this book and you should follow your doctor's advice. Good health follows from good nutrition. A rule of good nutrition is never to allow your fat storage to go above ten pounds, which is 35,000 calories in reserve.

3.
Protein and Amino Acids

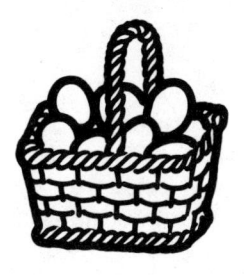

After energy, our second requirement from food is for protein. There are many kinds of proteins, and they are indispensable constituents of every living cell, making up more than half of all the organic material in our body. Just as the complex carbohydrate starch is built by a linking up of many smaller molecules of glucose, proteins are built by a linking up of many smaller molecules of amino acids. The amino acids, like glucose, are organic compounds made of linked up atoms of carbon, hydrogen, and oxygen, but they also contain nitrogen. Proteins contain carbon, hydrogen, oxygen, and nitrogen, but they also contain inorganic elements. Most contain sulphur and phosphorus; some contain iron, copper, and other minerals.

PROTEIN SOURCES AND FUNCTIONS

The food sources of protein are both plant and animal. Plants require proteins for their structure and life cycle. Just as they draw the elements they require for energy and carbohydrate synthesis from their environment, they draw the nitrogen they require from the soil, mainly as nitrates. But man and animals must get their protein-building material from food. Some animals eat only plant foods, some eat only other animals. Most people get their protein from both plant and animal sources. The familiar animal sources are eggs, milk, meat, and fish. The vegetable sources are all kinds of beans (for example, green beans, garbanzos, Indian grams, soybeans, navy beans, kidney beans); all kinds of peas and lentils; cereals (for example, oats, wheat, rye, millet, sorghum, corn); and peanuts and other nuts. Many other vegetables, from potatoes to leafy vegetables, contain amounts of protein that count when you add up the total eaten in a day.

Structural and Dynamic Material

You need proteins for the growth, maintenance, and repair of tissue and for the production of metabolic regulators and enzymes. They also supply the nitrogen needed for various other body constituents, particularly the nucleic acids so important in transmitting the characteristics of inheritance. Proteins perform indispensable functions in every living process.

The most easily understood and obvious function of protein is as the building material for all body tissues, such as muscle, heart, brains, kidney, liver, skin and hair.

But many other proteins have less obvious roles in the dynamic physiological exchanges of the life process. Each of the many blood proteins performs a specific function. Some carry nutrients to the cells; *hemoglobin* (the red cell protein) carries oxygen for metabolic reactions; *plasma* proteins maintain water balance and the slight alkalinity of the blood; other blood proteins cause clotting when the need arises; and protein *antibodies* maintain resistance to disease.

Enzymes are protein in nature and are catalysts for metabolic processes within the cell as well as for the breakdown of food in the digestive tract. *Hormones,* such as insulin, are the regulators of metabolic processes and many are protein. *Nucleoproteins* determine the pattern of inherited characteristics in the living cell.

An Energy Source

Energy is the first need of the body. If your food intake does not provide carbohydrates and fats or your body does not have fat stores to supply the energy required, body proteins will be broken down into amino acids. These amino acids will then be broken down further into compounds (similar to those from carbohydrate and fat) that are metabolized to energy, water, and carbon dioxide. When the amino acids are used for energy, they are reduced to their basic atoms and are lost as a source for protein synthesis.

Protein is also used as a source of energy when the intake of calories is adequate and the food intake of protein is greater than the body requirements. The amount of protein we require each day has undergone much study and is discussed more fully later in this chapter.

You need a daily supply of protein from food to replenish the amino acid pool so that the synthesis of body protein can equal the metabolic destruction. But once this amino acid need is met, any excess amino acids coming from the digestive tract are routed through the channels of either fat metabolism or carbohydrate metabolism to supply energy. If you are an active person, this energy is then used; if you are not active, it is stored as fat. There is no storehouse in the body for amino acids as such, nor are excess amino acids discarded in any way. The body is an extremely efficient metabolic plant. It merely alters the extra amino acids and stores them as fat to meet the body's primary need—energy.

The conversion of protein into fat is a wasteful process, both in terms of human obesity and the fattening of meat animals. The consumption of more protein does not make more muscle nor more meat.

A certain amount of protein is a source of energy each day through the channel of protein breakdown and the reduction of protein to amino acids again. Some of these are not reused for protein synthesis, but before being discarded their potential energy is used.

Protein Myths

In the days when we had much less knowledge of how the human body functions, it was easy to conclude that the proteins in food would have a direct relation to use in the body—for example, that red meat went to red blood and muscle formation, that gelatin from bones would make strong finger nails. But with the sophisticated methods we have today to study the workings of the living cell, we know that each plant, bird, fish, or animal synthesizes proteins that are uniquely its own. Each protein thus synthesized for its own use is patterned within the tissue cells for the cell's own specific needs. These proteins have specific structure; they are not interchangeable even within the same living creature.

A more recent misconception is that protein in cosmetic products has nourishment value. The fact that some proteins are soluble makes it possible to incorporate them into hair and skin cosmetics; but use of these products in no way contributes to the actual nourishment of the hair or skin because proteins are not absorbed into living cells this way. They may affect the appearance or surface, but they have no effect on the actual structure. They act much as starch in a collar—making the fabric stiff but not changing the fiber of the fabric.

AMINO ACIDS

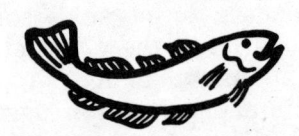

Proteins, like complex carbohydrates, are giant molecules built by linking hundreds and even thousands of smaller molecules. In the case of digestible carbohydrates, the small molecules are glucose. In the case of proteins the small molecules are amino acids.

There are 22 amino acids from which all proteins in nature, animal and plant, are made. From these 22 compounds your body is able to synthesize the hundreds of different proteins it needs for countless complex functions.

As we said at the beginning of the chapter, the amino acids, like glucose, are made up of atoms of carbon (C), hydrogen (H), and oxygen (O), with the characterizing difference of the addition of nitrogen (N) and sometimes sulphur (S). Another characteristic of amino acids is that they have a carboxyl (C-O-OH) group. The carbon (C) at one end of the chain is tightly bound to an oxygen (O) and a hydroxyl group (OH). This gives the amino acid the ability to react as an acid. The nitrogen (N), on the other hand, is bound to two hydrogens (H) as the amino group NH_2 and is attached to the next carbon in the chain. This gives the amino acid the ability to react as an alkaline.

Making Protein (Protein Synthesis)

When the amino acids are linked to form a protein, an amino group of one amino acid links to the carboxyl group of another, and a hydrogen and a hydroxyl group are split off. These unite to form water (H_2O). This happens at each bonding of amino acid to amino acid. The bond is called a *peptide bond*.

$$\text{amino acid 1} - \underset{\underset{H}{|}}{\overset{\overset{NH_2}{|}}{C}} - CO\boxed{OH + H}\underset{\underset{\text{amino acid 2}}{}}{\overset{\overset{H}{|}}{N}} - \overset{\overset{H}{|}}{\underset{\underset{}{|}}{C}} - COOH$$

$$\downarrow$$
$$H_2O$$
(water)

Hundreds and frequently thousands of amino acid molecules so linked make one protein molecule. Countless different protein patterns are possible, depending on the sequence and frequency of occurrence of specific amino acids. Protein structure also varies in how the molecules are linked. They can be a straight chain, folded in a coiled chain or helix, a branched chain, a hollow sphere, or a basket formation. Each combination, each variation in sequence, and each shape produces a protein with a specific character and function. It is rather like stringing beads, using 22 colors. If you run out of one color, you cannot make more strings of the same pattern.

Life Cycle of Protein

Each of the myriad proteins synthesized by the body cells is for their use. The life of many of them is very short. The structural proteins of body tissue (muscle, skin, organs, and cells) are ever-changing but relatively stable. The proteins that take part in physiological functions, (digestive enzymes), are constantly in the cyclical process of being synthesized, used for the purpose for which they were made, and in the process being split into amino acids again. These amino acids then become part of the amino acid pool and are free within the body cells, liver, and blood. The reuse of these amino acids to synthesize new protein is another amazing economy of protein metabolism. Even digestive enzymes used in the process of digesting food protein to the basic amino acids are absorbed along with the new ones and are available for resynthesis.

Synthesis Control

The control mechanism or "code" for the order and relationship of joining amino acids into proteins or protein synthesis is another substance containing nitrogen. The discovery of the factor that controls heredity within the gene was a key in unlocking how cells reproduce themselves. That factor or substance is deoxyribose nucleic acid, or DNA.

Proteins are synthesized in the cells in which they are to function. DNA ensures that the function of the cell remains essentially the same from one generation of them to the next. The DNA of the cell does not take part in protein synthesis directly but contains all the information or code necessary for it.

This whole process goes on quite rapidly, with a new protein being released in a matter of minutes. There must be an adequate supply of molecules of amino acids when the protein chain is being put together or the protein cannot be completed. Not only does the synthesis of protein depend on the presence of all the different amino acids needed for its structure, but they all must be there in sufficient quantities and at the same time.

For each one of the many reactions in this detailed picture of protein chemistry, a mineral, a vitamin, or another protein as an enzyme or hormone is needed to make it all happen. There may be more mysteries yet to uncover.

The tissue cell, in addition to protein synthesis, is able to make amino acids for its own protein-building function. However, the cells cannot make all 22 amino acids needed for protein-building—there are 8 needed by adults and 9 needed by children that cannot be synthesized and must be brought to the cell by the circulating blood. The blood picks them up from the digestive system, which has made them available from food.

Classification of Amino Acids

Amino acids are classified into two groups. Essential amino acids must be supplied daily by food. Nonessential amino acids need not come from food because the body can make them. Both groups are equally essential, however, for protein synthesis. Amino acids are also divided into groups depending on their structure, which in turn determines the part they play in living processes.

Biological Value (Quality) of Protein Foods

Based on the knowledge that for protein synthesis adults need eight amino acids and children nine, food proteins may

AMINO ACIDS

Group	Essential	Nonessential
Aliphatic: one amino, one carboxyl	Leucine Isoleucine Threonine Valine	Glycine Alanine Serine
Sulphur containing	Methionine	Cystine Cysteine
Basic: two amino, one hydroxyl	Lysine	Arginine Hydroxylysine

Acid: one amino, two hydroxyl		Aspartic acid
		Glutamic acid
		Hydroxy-
		  glutamic
		  acid

Cyclic	Tryptophan *Histidine	Proline Hydroxyproline
Aromatic	Phenyl- alanine	Tyrosine

NOTE: Two non-essential amino acids, cystine and tyrosine, reduce the need for two essential amino acids that they are like in structure. The presence of a good supply of cystine reduces the need for methionine, and tyrosine reduces the need for phenylalanine.

*Histidine is an essential amino acid for children; they need it to grow to their full potential. It has not been completely ruled out as an essential for adults in certain circumstances.

be divided into three groups, depending on which essential amino acids they contribute and the amount.

A food protein that contributes all eight or nine essential amino acids is called a *complete protein*. It will maintain body cells and promote growth. An *incomplete protein* is one that lacks one or more of the essential amino acids. It will not support life. A *partially complete* food protein is one that has an amino acid content that will maintain body cells but that fails to promote growth. The amino acid or acids that the incomplete or partially complete proteins lack is termed a *limiting amino acid*, because it limits the number of protein molecules that can be completed; if totally lacking, it prevents the entire protein synthesis.

The efficiency of the proteins of food in contributing to protein synthesis and thus to the overall physiological performance of the body has brought about a classification of protein foods based on biological function. The food that contributes the best balance of essential amino acids and best supply of nonessential amino acids for protein synthesis is the egg. This is understandable as it must supply all that is needed by the developing chick. For infants human milk outranks the egg. Such proteins are called *high quality*. The following chart shows familiar food sources of protein in decreasing order of biological value, or quality, based on growth studies.

QUALITY OF FAMILIAR FOOD PROTEINS

	*Average Serving	Protein grams	Biological Value %	Limiting Amino Acids
Egg	1	6	94	Complete
Milk	8 oz.	8	84	Complete
Fish	3½ oz.	28	83	Complete
Meat	3½ oz.	30	74	Complete
Soybeans	½ cup	10	73	Complete
Rice, brown	¾ cup	4	73	Incomplete: lysine, threonine
Whole wheat cereal	½ cup	2	65	Incomplete: lysine
Whole wheat dry cereal	¾ cup	2	65	Incomplete: lysine
Green leafy vegetables	½ cup	1–3	64	Incomplete: several amino acids
Rice, white	¾ cup	3	63	Incomplete: lysine, threonine
Potato	1 med.	3	60	Incomplete: several amino acids
Corn, whole grain	½ cup	3	59	Incomplete: lysine, tryptophan
Kidney beans	¾ cup	10	58	Incomplete: methionine
Peanut butter	1 Tbsp	4	54	Incomplete: several amino acids
Bread, white, wheat	1 slice	2	52	Incomplete: lysine

*Serving is for food as usually prepared.

The digestive process plays a very important role in subsequent protein synthesis from food proteins. In the digestive tract food proteins are reduced to their basic amino acids. As such they are then able to pass through the absorptive mechanism of the intestinal walls into the blood, then to the liver, and then, by means of the circulating blood, to the tissue cells. The mixture of foods eaten and digested and consequent mixture of amino acids absorbed is an important factor. Foods can supplement one another as sources of the amino acids for protein synthesis if they are eaten at the same meal.

Using Protein Foods That Supplement One Another

Combining foods that have complete proteins with those of incomplete proteins has resulted in many a fine dish, and the combination provides as much nutritional value as it does eating pleasure. It is a practice as old as time and seems to have been learned almost instinctively, or by observing how a people thrived or failed. Now that we have unlocked the chemistry, we know that many old favorites make the maximum use of the protein in each food; their combined amino acids are better able to meet the needs for protein synthesis. Examples are wheat, which lacks lysine, eaten with milk, which has an abundance; rice in combination with soybeans, for lysine and threonine; red beans and corn to supplement each other in lysine and methionine. All are mixtures in which the amino acids from one food make up for lacks or low levels of the other.

Time is also an important factor in protein synthesis. Protein synthesis is a rapid process when amino acids are present. Amino acids in excess of the balance needed to build protein are quite rapidly metabolized for energy. A synthesis process can be held up for four to six hours, but if the missing amino acid needed for the chain is not provided by then, the entire partially completed molecule is degraded.

This time factor makes it important to provide a good balance of amino acids by including some protein foods at each meal. Spacing the intake of complete protein foods throughout the day for maximum use of their amino acids seems more advantageous than eating a great amount in any single meal. So for maximum and efficient use of the protein foods, there should be a balance in each meal as well as each day.

On the surface it would appear that the lack of a certain

amino acid in a food could easily be made up by the addition of the synthetically produced amino acid—that pure crystalline lysine added to wheat cereal, for example, could take the place of milk as a source of lysine. In some instances where this has been tried, the results have been encouraging, but it has to be done with extreme care. Amino acids are antagonistic if they are out of balance. Too much of an amino acid can have as deleterious an effect as too little. If there is an excess of one amino acid, it may increase the need for or the use of others. Until we learn more about it, it is better to use foods that supplement one another.

End of Protein Cycle

When a protein has completed the use for which it was made, it is split into its component parts, not only amino acids but the other compounds with which it may have been joined. Sometimes these may be reused, but other times they are scheduled for destruction and excretion. When the amino acids from this breakdown or extra amino acids from food cannot be used for protein synthesis, they are changed chemically so they can enter the energy cycle at appropriate points.

The amino acids that are used to build body tissue yield no immediate energy, but once a cell discards an amino acid, it is finally metabolized. So it is a fallacy to think, "This protein food I am eating is going to build my body cells and is not a source of calories." It is a delayed source of calories. The body is superefficient with all its fuel sources, and amino acids no longer scheduled for protein synthesis will eventually be catabolized through the energy cycle for its energy and the urea cycle by which the nitrogen is excreted by the kidney.

Protein is the major substance used by the body that yields nitrogen as an end product, and it was by means of this excreted nitrogen that one method of determining protein requirement was developed.

How Protein Need Is Determined

In feeding experiments called balance studies, with human volunteers, different amounts and quality of proteins are fed and nitrogen excretion is calculated. As protein metabolism is the main source of this nitrogen, it is then possible to determine the nitrogen, thus protein, retained. On a low-protein diet, the excretion is greater than the supply, and the person is in "negative balance." On a high-protein diet, the excretion is less than the supply, showing that some was taken up in the tissues, and the person is in "positive balance." On a diet in which the intake and excretion are the same, the person is in "nitrogen equilibrium." The amount of protein needed for a healthy person to be in a state of equilibrium is the first determinant in calculating protein requirement.

Daily Requirement for Protein

The requirement for protein has changed upward and downward almost as many times as there have been investigators in the field. In any discussion of nutrient need, one must emphasize again and again that the science of nutrition is a new one, and that these changes are not whims or frauds but sincere beliefs based on new knowledge. The protein needs of the body have been studied longer than the needs of any other nutrient, but there are still differences of opinion.

The word *protein* was first used in 1838. In 1864 a researcher, Baron Justus von Liebig, published a book in which he stated that muscular work was done at the expense of protein structure—a concept that has advocates in athletic directors today. At the end of the 1800s the protein requirement for a man was considered to be about 118 grams per day; 145 grams for a man doing hard work. At the turn of the century, W. O. Atwater, one of America's nutrition pioneers, set the figure at 125 grams. Other researchers in the years following found that people could remain in nitrogen balance on as little as 40 grams.

Researchers also noted that the total energy level of the diet must be adequate in order for low levels of protein also to be adequate. When your diet is sufficiently high in carbohydrate and fats to meet the requirement for energy, then all the protein you eat is used to meet protein needs. A good level of carbohydrate in the diet is said to have a protein-sparing action. Fats also have a sparing action. So your daily protein requirement depends on the need for cell replacement (metabolic demands) and on the calories available from other foods and body fat.

In 1920 Henry Sherman completed a study, now considered

a classic, in which he determined that 44 grams of protein were needed for every 70 kilograms of body weight (1.5 ounces for 154 pounds).

In 1943 the National Academy of Sciences published the first Recommended Dietary Allowances of nutrients then known to be essential for optimum health. There was no need to set the figure for protein at the lowest level since extra protein in the diet would be used as energy. Because the foods eaten may vary in their balance of amino acids, a figure was chosen to allow a generous margin of safety. One gram of protein for each kilogram of body weight was the established daily recommended amount for adults.

In the next six editions of the RDA, 1 gram per kilogram of body weight for adults was still used even though during those same years much new knowledge was gained and the most desirable level of protein intake was still a question. In the eighth edition of 1874, the figure was lowered to almost that of Sherman's earlier studies.

Needs for protein are dependent on age, sex, and whether a woman is pregnant or breast-feeding her baby. Infants require the greatest amount of protein in relation to their body weight because infancy is the period of most rapid growth and adequate protein is vital for development and growth of the brain as well as the body. The average recommended allowance is 2.2 grams per kilogram of weight, but as infants aren't very big, their total protein need averages about 15 grams. The very best source is breast milk.

The recommended allowance for children 1 year old totals 23 grams. This increases each year as the child grows and is 36 grams for 10 year olds. The protein is needed for growth as well as daily cell replacement; every part of the body—bones, internal organs, muscles, and skin—is increasing in size.

Between the ages of 11 and 20, boys need more protein for growth and muscle development than girls. The increase for boys is from 36 to 54 grams, and for girls from 36 to 48 grams. After age 21 the average grown man has a recommended allowance of 56 grams of protein per day. Recent research has shown that the health and vigor of men past their sixties is best if this level of protein is maintained.

It is recommended that women maintain a protein intake of 46 grams daily, for their lifetime, except at those special times of pregnancy and breast-feeding. During pregnancy, a woman's protein need increases tremendously. In addition to her own needs of 46 grams, she needs 30 grams for her pregnancy, a total of 76 grams per day. For breast-feeding, the figures are 46 plus 20 for milk production, or 66 grams per day. It is vital that these needs be met for the perfect development of the baby, especially its brain. Pregnant teenagers have especially high protein needs because they must have enough for their own growth (48 grams) as well as for the high needs of pregnancy (30 grams). Chapter 13 presents foods for adults, infants, children, teenagers, pregnant women, and the elderly to meet protein requirements in balance with other essential nutrients.

Protein Deficiency

Protein deficiency diseases in nations that have inadequate food are protein-calorie deficiencies. One of these is *kwashiorkor*, a condition that results after weaning in children whose diet is mainly carbohydrates—sometimes at marginal levels. When a young child lacks protein for maintenance and growth, all the body stores of fat and muscle tissue are soon depleted and the life processes stop.

Reduction diets are not starvation diets, and they are very unlikely to result in a protein-deficiency condition. An overweight person would not develop a protein deficiency on a weight-loss regimen unless it were totally devoid of protein food. On the other hand, an excessively high-protein, low-calorie food intake can be a harmful way to lose weight because it can result in an imbalance of minerals.

4.
Minerals and Water

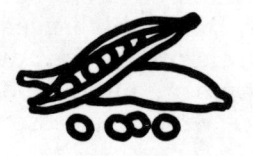

Carbohydrates, fats, and proteins are made of carbon, hydrogen, and oxygen, and they all supply energy. Protein, which also contains nitrogen and sometimes sulphur, supplies the amino acids for building material for muscles, soft tissue, skin, hair, etc. Carbohydrate, fat, and protein foods are called organic material because they are carbon compounds and come from other living animals or plants. Carbohydrate, fat containing linoleic acid, and the 9 essential amino acids are 11 of the almost 50 nutrients we know we need each day. In addition, we need other materials usually called minerals. These are inorganic material, and not minerals in the strictest sense of the word, but this is the simplest and most usual way to refer to them. The minerals we need in large amounts (100 milligrams or more each day) are called *major* or *macrominerals*. Minerals that we need in amounts of less than 100 milligrams, even as little as micrograms, are called *trace minerals*.

Control of Nutrient Transport by Minerals and Water

Water makes the whole of life possible. A person can live on stored fat, protein, and minerals for many months, but without water, life ends in a few days. Our bodies are about half water.

In very simple terms, our nutrition depends on nutrients being made soluble, then passing through membranes in three stages. Water carries the nutrients and oxygen as well as the various minerals that control how each nutrient passes along to where it is used. Water is also the medium by which the end products of nutrients are carried to points where they are excreted, or, in the case of carbon dioxide, exhaled.

We need about 1½ quarts of water each day. We get it from three sources. The first is by drinking water, plain or in the form of soup or beverages. The second is from foods high in water—fruits, vegetables, and milk, for example. The third is from glucose and fats which produce water in the cell when they are converted to energy.

MACROMINERALS

The macrominerals are calcium, phosphorus, magnesium, sodium, potassium, chlorine (as chloride), and sulphur.

Calcium and Phosphorus

Of all the minerals, we require calcium and phosphorus in the greatest amounts because they are the major materials of our skeleton and teeth. Our whole bodily appearance depends on how well our bones and teeth are formed. Our adult appearance depends on our getting an adequate daily intake of calcium throughout the rest of our lives. Bones and teeth, living tissue built of protein and minerals, are constantly exchanging old material for new. About one-third of bone is a protein structure, or matrix, made of collagen. You can think of it as a sponge with regularly shaped holes throughout. The holes are filled with calcium and phosphorus in almost equal amounts, as crystals of calcium phosphate which make the bone strong. Bone also contains some calcium carbonate, small amounts of magnesium, and fluorine, a trace mineral. The process is called *mineralization*. The exterior of bone and teeth, especially the enamel, is more compactly mineralized than the interior. The more porous interior makes the exchange of elements with the blood supply in the protein sponge possible.

The bones act as storage depots for calcium, phosphorus, and magnesium, and are constantly drawn on for bodily functions. The level of these minerals, and the ratio between them in the food you eat daily, affects the amount withdrawn or deposited. Once the enamel of the teeth is formed, however, it is practically unchanged by the level of calcium in the diet. Vitamin D is another nutrient vital for proper bone and tooth formation. It promotes the absorption of calcium from the digestive system, and also acts in depositing the calcium in the protein matrix. Two other nutrients, vitamins A and C (ascorbic acid), are needed in the development of the matrix. Vitamin D can be made from a form of cholesterol present in the skin, when the skin is exposed to sunshine. The growth and health of bones and teeth are a clear example of how the functions of nutrients are interrelated.

About 99 percent of your body calcium is in your bones and teeth and about 1 percent is in the body fluids. About 700 milligrams of calcium enter and leave your bones every day, and about 320 milligrams of this calcium, after performing metabolic uses in your body fluids, is lost by excretion. The calcium level in the blood and the fluids of the body tissues is kept at a constant level. The proper balance between calcium, phosphorus, and magnesium in the fluid around the heart is responsible for its normal rhythmic beating. The calcium in the blood is essential for blood clotting. It is responsible for nerve transmission and the normal tone and reaction of muscles. It also activates enzymes in the release of energy.

Calcium does not act alone, but seems to be the coordinator of other minerals. All the organs controlled by the central nervous system depend on the presence of calcium, phosphorus, magnesium, and sodium in just the right proportions. For all bodily functions to proceed normally, the level of all mineral salts in blood and tissues is kept at a constant level and in proper balance, chiefly by hormones.

Calcium and Growth

Our need for calcium is greatest in relationship to our body weight when we are infants. Under the influence of growth hormones, the protein part of the bone grows, and the diet must provide enough calcium to mineralize it and make it strong. A high-protein, low-calcium diet only provides part of the needs for bone building. At certain ages growth is rapid.

The first period of rapid growth is the first year, when a baby's needs are best supplied by breast milk. Formula milk may have a higher calcium content but the baby absorbs and retains less of this calcium. The rate of growth slows after the first year, but the calcium need between the ages of two and three remains high per pound of body weight as the new bone is more calcified. During these years, the enamel of the permanent teeth is almost completely mineralized. Children from two to ten require two to four times as much calcium per pound of body weight as adults do. The Recommended Dietary Allowance is set at 800 milligrams per day, which allows a liberal margin of safety. The next most rapid and the final growth period is adolescence. At this time the need goes up to 1000 to 1200 milligrams (1 to 1.2 grams) per day. Children and teenagers are more prone to cavities than adults. During the growth years, teeth continue to mature and their roots continue to grow. After your time of growth, if your adult weight is about 120 pounds and your bones are well mineralized, they will contain 1300 grams or about 3 pounds of calcium.

Calcium in Adult Years

The RDA for adults is 800 milligrams, which is more than adequate to cover the 300 milligrams or so lost each day and to allow a margin of safety, since only about 40 percent of the calcium in your diet is absorbed. It also allows a margin of safety for persons who have a high protein intake since studies have shown their calcium losses can be substantial.

The greatest need of women for calcium is during pregnancy and breast-feeding. The developing baby draws on its mother's bone calcium before it is born, so the mother must be sure to balance this withdrawal. Then later she needs extra calcium to provide for the calcium in her milk. Before the baby is born, both its baby and permanent teeth are formed, and the baby teeth are almost completely calcified. During pregnancy and breast-feeding the RDA is the same as during adolescence (1200 milligrams or 1.2 grams). The pregnant teenager who has not completely grown nor mineralized bones is at a great disadvantage from both calcium and protein needs. She needs at least 1000 milligrams for herself and an additional 400 for pregnancy, or a total of 1400 to 1600 milligrams (1.4 to 1.6 grams) per day. (See RDA table, page 97.)

Deficiencies

Rickets: A Childhood Bone Problem

Rickets is a condition of poor bone formation resulting from deficiencies of calcium and vitamin D. Bowed-out leg bones are the overt result. When a child with poorly mineralized bones starts to walk the bones become permanently bent out of shape. There are other less obvious poorly formed bones as well. Since the discovery of vitamin D, rickets has rarely been seen in this country. Cod liver oil, a potent source, was regularly prescribed for infants and children, and subsequently milk was fortified with vitamin D. Rickets can reappear, however, if babies are not fed foods that supply their needs for minerals and are not given vitamin D supplements.

Osteomalacia: Adult Form of Rickets

Adult vitamin D deficiency is not a common condition in this country since we are sun worshippers. But osteomalacia can occur in pregnancy and among persons who get little sunlight and take no form of vitamin D.

Osteoporosis: Possible Calcium Deficiency

At the other end of the age span from infantile rickets is osteoporosis, a condition in which the bones become thin and break easily. This condition may be the result of the generally held idea that once bones are formed they remain unchanging. We now know that adults need to maintain a constant calcium intake to keep their bones strong for their lifetime. The RDA of 800 milligrams allows a margin of safety for decreased absorption as one gets older. In osteoporosis, however, there are also changes in the bone matrix. Adequate protein is needed, as well as vitamins A and C, for maintaining the base structure.

In the last 15 years milk consumption among adults has decreased, and protein, especially meat consumption, has increased. The higher the protein in the diet the greater the calcium loss. Another dietary change has been the drinking of soft drinks instead of water, many of which contain phosphoric acid. Calcium absorption is affected by the ratio of calcium to phosphorus, and the result of these changes has been an imbalanced calcium-to-phosphorus intake ratio of almost 1:4. Although the ideal ratio is 1:1 or 1:2 vitamin D has some protective effect at high phosphorus ratios.

The loss of calcium sneaks up on us, and if your diet is corrected in time, you may possibly avoid such consequences as the broken hip so often suffered by elderly women. Men are less prone to severe bone loss, as they usually have larger bone mass. Small women who have small bones are the most prone. The first evidence of bone loss is in the jaw; this can be detected by your dentist when he X-rays your teeth. You should ask him if you are developing a warning sign, periodontal disease. The loss of calcium may be responsible for resorbed or fractured vertebrae, the appearance of the "dowager hump."

Hormones also play a role as yet not fully understood in the loss of calcium from bone. Not all persons have bone problems as they get older. Some elderly do not develop fractures but become shorter.

Some persons are better able to conserve calcium stores as well as to absorb it better from foods. But if you choose foods that supply you with adequate calcium and vitamins A and C, you will be doing much to keep your bones in good health.

Needs for Phosphorus

About 80 percent of your body's phosphorus is in your bones and teeth. The other 20 percent is in the soft tissues and organs and in every cell. In contrast to calcium, which is relatively inert, phosphorus is very reactive. It can combine in many ways with many substances, transporting them in blood and body fluids, depositing some and picking up others. It plays a part in keeping the blood neutral by combining with alkaline substances produced by cell function. It also combines with fats and fatty acids and transports them to where they are needed or stored. It sparks the energy release from carbohydrate as a part of several of the enzymes involved in this series of reactions. It has an essential role in protein synthesis within the cell. It is the most active mineral substance in the body and is involved in almost every metabolic process.

There is little chance of having a phosphorus deficiency, because it is in so many foods. It is so prevalent that the Committee on Dietary Allowances did not feel it necessary to make a recommendation for phosphorus until the 1974 edition, when an amount equal to the RDA for calcium was established. This was made more as a balance to calcium intake than to define a need for phosphorus.

In the preceding section we discussed the calcium-to-phosphorus ratio in relation to the health of bones when too little calcium is available. Too much phosphorus can have the same effect. One of the food sources of phosphorus is protein. A high protein diet is an acid-producing one, as the phosphorus, the sulphur, and the carbon chains of proteins, when metabolized, all produce acid end products (phosphoric, sulphuric, and carbonic acids). They require basic substances to buffer or neutralize them. Neutralizing minerals are calcium, sodium, potassium, and magnesium. An unbalanced calcium-to-phosphorus ratio in your food also results in an imbalance in the amount of each that is absorbed and can have the same effect as low calcium intake.

It is easier for your body to maintain a calcium-and-phosphorus balance as well as an acid-and-base balance if the foods you eat are similarly closely balanced.

Six Common Errors in Eating Habits That May Lead to Bone Problems When You Get Older

- Not eating foods that supply the 800 milligrams of calcium you need daily. (Our best source of calcium is milk or unsweetened milk products.)
- Eating more food than you need and accumulating extra weight as fat which your bones have to support.
- Disregarding calcium needs and avoiding needed protective foods out of fear of gaining too much weight, when you are young.
- Drinking phosphoric acid drinks (such as soda pop) instead of natural hard water or scientifically fluoridated water.
- Following poorly conceived and improperly balanced reduction diets to reduce fat weight, especially high-protein regimens and low-carbohydrate fad diets.
- Not getting the calcium needed during pregnancy, especially if you are a teenager.

Magnesium

Our need for calcium and phosphorus was known as long ago as 1900, but it wasn't until 1933 that our positive need for magnesium was verified and not until 1964 that it was included as a dietary essential in the Recommended Dietary Allowances (RDA).

Like calcium, magnesium is essential for bone structure. It is stored in bones and plays an active role in body cells. Your body contains about 25 grams of magnesium, of which half is in your bones. The other half is in the cells of muscle and liver. In the cells, it activates the enzymes that release energy from blood sugar (glucose). In plant life, magnesium in the green chlorophyll is responsible for trapping the sun's energy in the form of glucose.

Magnesium is essential within the cell for the synthesis of protein. It has a part in the working of muscles and nerves and in the regulation of body temperature. Our absorption of magnesium from food depends on the levels of calcium, protein, phosphorus, and vitamin D in our diet. It is widely available in whole grain cereals and leafy vegetables, and milk is a fairly good source; thus a deficiency has been considered most unlikely. However, processing can lower the magnesium content of foods considerably. Refining cereals and oils removes almost all their magnesium, and the two-time cooking or heating of "convenience" vegetables also results in losses.

People most likely to show a deficiency of magnesium are those who eat no whole grain cereals and few vegetables. Alcoholics, who have an increased loss of magnesium and usually a poor food intake, frequently show magnesium deficiency.

Sulphur

One macromineral we get in organic but not in mineral form is sulphur. We get it bound in protein in the essential amino acid methionine and also in the amino acid cysteine, which can be converted to methionine. Sulphur is an essential part of both vitamin B_1 (thiamin) and biotin. It is also needed for insulin, a hormone that regulates glucose metabolism, and for glutathione, another metabolic regulator. Thiamin is a coenzyme also involved in the release of energy from glucose.

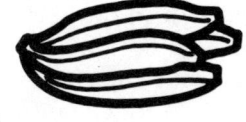

Sodium, Potassium, and Chloride

In general, these elements occur in combined form as salts such as sodium chloride or potassium chloride. Our first need for chloride is in the digestive process in the stomach, where water and chloride are combined as hydrochloric acid. The first stage of nutrition is digestion; all the foods we eat are reduced to nutrients in solution in the digestive juices. In order to understand the role of sodium, potassium, and chloride (called electrolytes), you need to review certain physiological processes.

After digestion in the stomach, the process continues in the small intestine, where other digestive juices, enzymes, and salts come into action. In the normal healthy person all these stages and those following are regulated by hormones to keep the proper balance and level of nutrients and minerals for all cells to function normally. The first membranes the nutrients have to pass through are the walls of the digestive tract, where the blood picks up what the body requires. Then the blood goes to the liver, and some of the nutrients are processed into more available forms for the cells and returned to the blood. The blood circulates in the body, and the nutrients pass through the membranes or walls of the blood system and into the extracellular fluid around the cells. Through their cell membranes, each individual cell takes from this fluid what it requires to rebuild its structure and/or produce energy.

All these exchanges are under the control of the macrominerals. Concentrations of sodium, potassium, and chloride are the regulators for the passage of nutrients in and out of the cells. The process is tremendously complicated. Once again, the most important factor is balance. When too much or too little of some salt is taken in, it upsets the balance. Sodium works outside the cell; with chloride, it regulates body fluid volume. Potassium works inside the cell and is necessary for protein and carbohydrate metabolism.

There is little likelihood that you will have a lack of these three elements in your diet. In the case of sodium chloride (table salt) we may use too much. A continuous use of too much table salt can result in high blood pressure. When doctors recommend a decrease in salt to alleviate this condition, it is sodium they wish decreased, so you must read the ingredient listing on food packages for all mention of sodium, not just of sodium chloride.

For other conditions, a doctor may recommend orange juice to increase potassium intake. Be aware that while natural orange juice is an excellent source of potassium, orange-flavored drinks with a high vitamin C content are not.

Because there is no lack of sodium, potassium, and chloride in our wide food selection, there is no RDA for persons in good health. (Specific recommendations for certain disease conditions are not within the scope of this book.) Again, we can correct errors in our present lifestyle—one of which is the error of eating high-protein and high-salt snack foods.

- High protein snack foods draw on alkaline and calcium reserves.
- High-salt snack foods require the elimination of the extra sodium from the body and make more work for the kidneys.

If you snack on fruits instead, they will provide fewer calories and more water; they are alkaline in reaction and provide minerals in amounts that do not unbalance the system.

TRACE MINERALS

Because trace minerals are present in such minute amounts in our bodies, our understanding of the roles and of our needs for these has required long and tedious research. There are seven minerals we know we need in trace amounts for our bodies to function in perfect health. There are at least another seven found in our tissues that we can assume we need since they are there; but as yet we don't know exactly why we need them. And there may be many more that are still eluding nutrition researchers. Some of the first seven have been known since recorded medical history. The knowledge of the next seven has been learned in just the last few years. Using the latest techniques, research on these and others is one of the most active areas in the nutrition field today.

On a food intake of fresh and traditionally cooked foods, it is unlikely that you will develop a deficiency of the trace minerals. But as more food is processed and sequestrants are used to inactivate or bind these minerals in order to give packaged products a long shelf life, it is possible that people who use a lot of such products might develop a lack of one or more trace minerals.

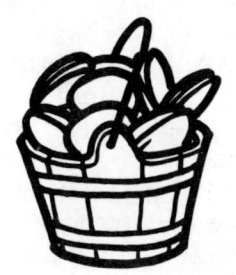

Iodine

The oldest known essential mineral is iodine. The existence of a substance in seaweed that had a specific beneficial effect on health was known 5000 years ago in the Orient. The substance, iodine, was found to prevent goiter, an enlargement of the thyroid gland. Iodine has only one function. It is an integral part of the hormones produced in the thyroid gland. Thyroxine is the hormone that sets the pace of basal metabolism, and it is vital for normal growth from conception to adulthood. In simple terms, basal metabolism is the base rate at which your body uses energy to exist while at rest, that is, for the life-sustaining work of the heart, lungs, organs, digestive tract, and so forth. When there isn't enough iodine available, the thyroid gland becomes enlarged in its effort to make enough hormones for your body's need.

Goiter has been prevalent in all parts of the world since recorded history. Despite our present-day knowledge it is still one of the most prevalent world health problems. Iodine deficiency occurs in areas where there is little or no iodine in the soil or rainfall, and in isolated inland areas, where foods from the sea are not available. The oceans are vast reservoirs of iodine, and seafood is rich in iodine. Persons living in coastal regions get their supply from ocean fish as well as from the rain that falls on their vegetables and water supply.

That iodine was the element in seaweed that prevented the development of goiter was discovered in the early nineteenth century. Nearly a hundred years (1914) after it was found that iodine was the essential element in the hormones produced by the thyroid gland, a simple solution to goiter was introduced by adding iodine to table salt. In most countries this is one of the simplest and cheapest ways of eliminating a still-prevalent deficiency disease.

The thyroid hormones are essential for growth, so they are vital for the normal development of babies before and after birth. A lack of iodine not only affects physical development but retards mental development. Babies born of mothers deficient in iodine are most likely to be cretins. With such a simple solution as adding iodine to table salt one would think that goiter and cretinism would have been eradicated by now. Instead, there is some evidence that goiter is increasing even in the United States. This may be due to the misconception that iodized salt has an "additive" rather than a nutrient put in it. Another reason may be that since it is not mandatory that iodized salt be used in manufactured products, most products do not contain iodized salt.

The salt intake of Americans comes from "convenience" and snack foods more now than it did ten years ago. Switzerland and Canada require that all salt used in processing foods and all table salt be iodized. The Food and Nutrition Board has recommended that federal legislation be enacted in the United States to make iodization of food salt mandatory. Because the elimination of iodine deficiency disease has not been as sure and simple a thing as might have been expected, an RDA for iodine was established in 1968. The amount needed for various ages is shown in the RDA Table on page 97. Remember, you can get all you need by using moderate amounts of iodized salt.

Thyroid health and function used to be determined by checking basal metabolic rate (BMR), the consumption of oxygen for metabolic functions. Now your doctor uses a simple blood test for protein-bound iodine (PBI).

Iron

Iron, essential for red blood cells, was known as a vital mineral to doctors in ancient Greece. Yet it remains the trace mineral most lacking in the American diet today. Our consumption of refined foods is one of the reasons. A fair percent of our population have iron deficiency anemia, the commonest form of iron deficiency.

Iron is a constituent of your blood. About 70 percent of it is in the hemoglobin of the red blood cells, where it gives them the ability to pick up oxygen in your lungs and transport it to the cells, where it is used to release energy. Then the iron in the hemoglobin combines with the carbon dioxide produced by the process and carries it to the lungs, where it is released and exhaled. If you have an iron deficiency, your red blood cells are smaller than normal and do not have a full supply of hemoglobin. They cannot pick up the proper amount of oxygen in your lungs to supply the cells with all they need to function. You are always tired, easily worn out, sometimes have headaches or get short of breath on exertion, and are usually pale. Your blood has a reduced capacity for carrying oxygen to cells and for removing carbon dioxide from the cells to the lungs to be exhaled. One of the simplest and most frequently used diagnostic tests shows the level of hemoglobin in the blood. Don't do self-diagnosis from the above symptoms; they could also come from other conditions. Have your hemoglobin level checked by your doctor.

The life span of a red blood cell is about 120 days. Some cells are always being made, and old worn-out cells are discarded. The 30 percent of the iron not in red blood cells is in the liver, spleen, and bone marrow, where it is available for making new red blood cells. And a small percent is in the tissues and cells, where it is needed for the life process.

When old red blood cells are biodegraded, your body has a great ability to save the iron. But some is lost each day, so you need some daily replacement. Some circumstances increase your need for iron. Children need more as they grow and develop a larger blood supply. Teenagers need extra for their growth spurt, especially girls who also start having menstrual losses. There is a greatly increased need for iron during pregnancy, both for the mother and the developing baby. The loss of blood through injury also results in loss of iron. If you are a blood donor, you must watch your diet. And if you are trying to lose weight and are counting calories and not counting iron, you could become anemic as well as thin.

Whenever you have an increased need for iron, your body adapts to absorb more from your food. But if the iron is not in the food, then deficiency will result. Iron is best absorbed when it has been freed from organic material and is in the acid area of digestion. The iron of liver, eggs, and muscle meat is readily used after digestion of these foods. The iron of green vegetables is well absorbed, especially if they also contain a good amount of vitamin C (ascorbic acid). The iron in whole grain cereals is bound to phosphates or phytates, but can be absorbed. As is the case with other minerals, iron in excess amounts may be toxic.

There are other complicated (and sometimes disease) conditions that affect iron absorption, so even though men and post-menstrual women only lose about 1 milligram each day, their requirement is set at almost ten times that amount. Iron requirements are shown for each age group in the RDA table on page 97. Liver is the best food source of iron, and next best are eggs, meats, leafy green vegetables, molasses, dried beans (even better when cooked with molasses), apricots, raisins, and whole grain and enriched cereals and breads.

Copper

It wasn't until the 1930s that copper was also found to be important in blood formation. By this time, quite a number of nutrients had been partially isolated, and it was possible to prepare experimental diets that were adequate enough to keep animals alive yet refined enough to show cause and effect of adding and subtracting small amounts of materials. Continued study has shown that copper plays a part in the absorption and use of iron for the formation of hemoglobin. Copper is found in all body tissues, especially in the brain and vital organs. It plays many metabolic roles.

Copper, present in many foods, is one of the elements that affects the shelf life of packaged foods; if sequestered, it may be poorly absorbed. Sometimes it is removed in processing, so the copper content of refined foods is questionable. No RDAs have been established, but by eating traditional foods you get an adequate copper supply from liver and muscle meats, shellfish, dried beans, and cocoa.

Cobalt

Cobalt is another trace element involved in the process of blood formation. It is used only as a part of the vitamin B_{12} molecule. Cobalt is like sulphur in that it is supplied in an already formed essential compound. A deficiency of vitamin B_{12} results in nutritional anemias, which are discussed under the B-vitamins.

Manganese and Zinc

Two trace elements, manganese and zinc, are essential for the intricate enzyme system of cell metabolism. Manganese deficiency can be produced in experimental animals, but it is unlikely to occur in humans. Manganese is present in many foods but, like the other trace minerals, can be affected by processing. Nuts and whole grains are excellent sources. Meat contains little. Manganese is a catalyst in cell processes and is present in enzymes. It is needed in the use of glucose for energy, in the making of fats for storage and of cholesterol for the nerve system, and for the normal working of muscles. It is present in bone and vital organs. How it performs all its vital functions is still a matter of study and fascination. No RDAs have been established.

Zinc is present in insulin and is involved in the production and function of other hormones. It plays an active role in the cells in protein synthesis, especially the proteins of skin and collagen. In the enzyme system, by which energy is released from glucose in the cells, the role of zinc is the removal of carbon dioxide.

Zinc deficiency was considered unlikely until it showed up in persons following restricted vegetarian diets. Zinc is prevalent in many plant and animal foods, but it is lost in refining. A deficiency is most unlikely to develop if you eat a wide selection of fresh foods, including milk, meat, eggs, and whole grains. A zinc deficiency can upset the intricate functions mentioned above. As in any such deficiency, normal growth and development suffer. Zinc deficiency as seen and diagnosed in the Middle East results in dwarfism.

Recent evidence of the existence of marginal zinc intake levels in segments of our population led to the establishment in 1974 of RDAs for zinc (table, page 97).

Fluorine

Fluorine, a vital element in teeth and bone formation, functions alongside calcium, phosphorus, and magnesium. Fluorine is present in differing amounts in the many lakes and rivers of the country. In areas where it was present in high levels in the water, it was found to cause brown marks on the teeth of children who grew up drinking such water. Despite the brown marks, the teeth of these children were very resistant to caries. Fluorine is now removed from drinking water in these areas. But it was learned that even very low levels of fluorine in water or diet makes the calcium crystals of bone and especially teeth more stable.

As with the other trace elements, the complete role of fluorine is still being studied. It seems possible that an adequate fluorine intake may benefit the elderly in regard to bone loss, just as it benefits the young in the development of strong tooth enamel. Some studies have shown decreased occurrence of bone loss in older persons who live where water is fluoridated. No RDAs have been established, but fluoridation of the drinking water is done in the United States and other countries where the fluorine content is low. Fluorine, like iodine, is present in ocean fish and seafood. Tea is another good source.

Trace Elements Under Study

Seven more trace elements have been isolated from human cells. From their presence, we can infer a function. Experiments done with animals may lead us to the answers, but it is very poor science to assume that humans will react as laboratory animals do. Consequently you should be wary of articles that hail miracles and the discovery of the elixir of youth by reporting out of context serious work on these elements.

1. *Molybdenum:* In 1953 this element was found to be a component of xanthine dehydrogenase, one of our essential enzymes.
2. *Selenium:* In 1957 the importance of selenium to animals was determined. It is very closely related to the function of vitamin E and seems to "spare" vitamin E. Selenium is an antioxidant and protects cell membranes. It is toxic in large amounts and the first studies done on it were as a mineral in the soil, toxic to farm animals.
3. *Chromium:* In 1959 it was established that chromium was essential to man as well as to animals. Several functions, all at the enzyme level, have been discovered. Chromium is required for the release of energy from glucose, probably as part of the hormone insulin. It has roles in other enzyme systems too; one system is the production of fatty acids and cholesterol and another system is the digestion of protein. No specific requirement has yet been determined, but evidence points to a greater need by pregnant women and older persons. Chromium is removed from refined foods.
4. *Nickel:* In 1970 a nickel deficiency was observed in chickens. Nickel is probably essential for us. Its role seems to be in the making of hormones and some proteins.
5. *Tin:* In 1970 the need for tin in the synthesis of protein was seen in rats. Our need for tin is no doubt met by canned foods, since most cans have tin linings.
6. *Vanadium:* In 1971 vanadium was added to the list of trace elements that are probably essential. It is a catalyst in several living processes, one being the mineralization of teeth. We are not likely to have a deficiency, since it is very difficult even to devise an experimental deficient diet.
7. *Silicon:* In 1972, rats' need for silicon was shown. It is needed for the normal development of the cartilage matrix in bone. But silicon is the most abundant mineral on earth; as sand, there is no lack of it. Silicon is widely distributed in foods.

One final word must be said about the trace elements. We require them in minute (trace) amounts. Many of them can be toxic if too much is taken for too long a time. Fluorine's relationship to brown mottled teeth is the most obvious example. The trace elements work in balance together. Too much of one can unbalance others enough to cause a deficiency.

5.
Vitamins

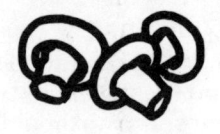

Vitamins are organic rather than mineral substances. They are made of the same basic elements, carbon, hydrogen, and oxygen, as carbohydrates, fats, and proteins. Their structure is more complicated, however, and some have nitrogen or a mineral element incorporated in them. Vitamin B_{12}, for example, has cobalt. Vitamins do not supply us with energy. Nor are they part of our body structure as the minerals and protein are. The part vitamins play in our bodies is to bring about the chemical reactions of the process of life. Vitamins are catalysts, substances that cause reactions to occur. In living plants and animals, catalysts are referred to as enzymes. Sometimes enzymes themselves require a catalyst, which is called a coenzyme.

Each vitamin causes specific reactions to happen, ranging from the constant release of energy from glucose to the clotting of blood when you prick your finger. Yet for all the hundreds of reactions they bring about, they are needed in relatively small amounts. Enzymes are not used up in the reactions they spark; they are released and can be used again and again, eventually being replaced by new ones. So only small amounts of the vitamins are used up and need to be replaced each day. Their function as a part of many enzymes is one of two things all the vitamins have in common. The other is that we must get our daily supply from food. We cannot synthesize or make vitamins in our bodies. In this respect they are like the essential amino acids.

The term *vitamin* was coined in 1912 by a Dr. Funk, who

thought that the factors in foods that cured deficiency diseases were "vital amines," shortened over the years to vitamin. The substance he was working on turned out to be thiamin(e), the only amine of the vitamins. It is unfortunate that vitamins are promoted as curative substances to such a degree in popular writing. It is true that the early research was concerned with finding the curative factors for such conditions as rickets, scurvy, beriberi, pellagra, and xerophthalmia. But now that these conditions have all but been eliminated in this country we know the vitamins are preventive factors—nutrients that prevent these conditions from developing. We should think of vitamins as nutrients in food that promote and protect our overall good health. In the well-fed nations of the world today, the severe deficiency diseases of old are rarely seen. But in many parts of the world, despite present knowledge, deficiency diseases are a major problem.

As the knowledge of the vitamins unfolded, the first to be isolated as the unknown factor in a food having a beneficial effect was logically named "A." Others were discovered and were named by other letters—B, C, D, and so forth. However, it was soon found that vitamin B was a complex of several vitamins, so the lettering system broke down. In the last few years the precise chemistry of the vitamins has been determined, so they now have names that are based on their chemical structure. A list of the known vitamins with their old and new names to sort out the confusion follows.

The vitamins are divided into two groups, depending on their solubility. Vitamins A, D, E, and K are fat soluble. They are found in the fat or oil of foods. In order for them to be absorbed during digestion, there must be some fat or oil in the meal. They are all stored to some extent in your body. The B-complex vitamins and vitamin C are water soluble. This makes them more easily lost when foods are cooked in water. They are not stored in your body, and any extra consumed beyond your body's need is excreted.

In the course of research on the water-soluble vitamins many factors were found and named in different labs and countries. They have now been identified as being the same as some vitamins, while some factors have been proven to have no nutritional value. Among the outmoded names are vitamin G, vitamin H, vitamin M, vitamin P, vitamin B_{10}, vitamin B_{15}, vitamin B_{17}, factor L, factor R, factor U, bioflavinoids, hesperidin, and rutin.

Vitamin	Old Name	New Name
Vitamin A		Retinol
Vitamin B	B-complex:	
	vitamin B_1	Thiamin
	vitamin B_2	Riboflavin
	pellagra preventative (nicotinic acid)	Niacin
	vitamin B_6	Pyridoxine
		Pantothenic acid
	Folic acid	Folacin
	vitamin B_{12}	Cyanocobalamine
		Biotin
		Choline
Vitamin C	Antiscorbutic	Ascorbic acid
Vitamin D	Antirachitic	
Vitamin D_2		Calciferol
Vitamin D_3		25-hydroxy-cholecalciferol
Vitamin E		Alpha-tocopherol
Vitamin K		Menaquinone
Vitamin K_3 (synthetic form)		

FAT-SOLUBLE VITAMINS

Vitamin A

Extreme vitamin A deficiency is currently one of the world's most serious health problems. It is the Third World's most serious and most prevalent deficiency disease. The condition is xerophthalmia. It begins as night blindness, then progresses to degenerative changes in the eye that result in permanent blindness. This degree of deficiency is not a problem in countries with a good supply of milk, eggs, and certain fruits and vegetables. It can be cured in the early stages by therapeutic doses of vitamin A. It can be prevented by an adequate diet. Vitamin A is added to our skim milk and margarine to ensure us a sufficient supply of vitamin A.

Functions of Vitamin A

Vitamin A is vital for healthy eyes and normal vision. The role vitamin A plays in vision is in the retina or part of the eye which reacts to light. We see light and dark and colors by changes in the surface of the retina. Vitamin A (retinol) restores the surface after each reaction. If you don't have an adequate supply of vitamin A to do this, the restoration is slow and your eyes do not adapt quickly to changes from light to dark. You will have poor vision when you go into a dark room, not be able to see well when driving a car at dusk, or be momentarily blinded by oncoming passing headlights. These are symptoms of night blindness.

Vitamin A is involved in keeping all our exposed surfaces healthy—our exterior skin and the interior linings of our mouth, eyes, ears, and our breathing, digestive, urinary, and other systems. When these surfaces, or *epithelial tissues*, are in the best of health, your skin is smooth and soft; and when the interior tissues are healthy, they are moist and have a high resistance to infection. This is especially true of the linings of the throat and most important in the tear glands and moist tissue that surrounds your eyes.

Vitamin A is essential for normal growth. A function of almost every vitamin is stimulation of normal growth, since vitamins are involved in the use of all the other nutrients. Vitamin A plays a role in the development of the bone matrix as a child's skeleton increases in all dimensions to adult size. In the grown adult, vitamin A may play a part in the continued health of the protein part of bone. Vitamin A also has a role in the reproductive cycle and the production of hormones.

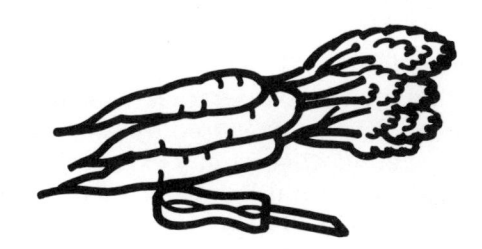

Sources of Vitamin A

We get vitamin A from plant and animal foods. The most concentrated source is fish liver oils, which are used in vitamin supplements and in fortifying margarine and skim milk. Although some are fortified with synthetic retinol plus carotene, they can be counted as animal food sources. Other animal sources are liver, egg yolk, butter, milk, and cheese.

The plant sources of vitamin A are carotenes which can be converted to vitamin A during the digestive process. They are called provitamins. Plant foods high in carotene are deep yellow in color—carrots, winter squash, sweet potatoes, pumpkin, apricots, peaches. Tomatoes and green leafy vegetables are also sources of carotene. Carotene is not affected adversely by heat. In fact, because we digest cooked vegetables better than raw ones, we get more potential vitamin A when they are cooked.

Vitamin A from all sources is better absorbed when there is some fat or oil in the meal.

Mineral oil is not a food oil. It prevents the absorption of vitamin A, so it should never be used as a calorie-free oil in cooking or salad dressings. Mineral oil should be used only on your doctor's advice.

The vitamin A content of foods is most usually given in International Units (IU). An International Unit is a measure of vitamin A activity in reversing deficiency symptoms (established in 1934).

How Much We Need

Because one of the functions of vitamin A is to aid in the growth of bones and the development of teeth, infants, children, and teenagers need more than adults. Requirements for infants are based on body weight; but by the age of one, the average baby needs 2000 IU. Between the ages of one and eleven, as children grow, the need increases until it reaches the adult requirement of 5000 IU for boys and 4000 IU for girls. During pregnancy, women need an additional 1000 IU and 1000 IU more if they breast-feed their baby. (See RDA table, page 96.)

Can we get too much vitamin A? Vitamin A is one of the vitamins that is stored in our bodies, mainly in the liver. This is an advantage as any extra taken in over what is needed daily to replace what has been used is retained and used when your food intake is below your requirement. Since deficiencies do not happen suddenly, you usually have enough stored so that you need to review your vitamin A intake only on a week-to-week basis. Storage of vitamin A is a disadvantage for persons who take large amounts in capsule form. Too much produces a toxic condition, or hypervitaminosis A. This has been observed in children more often than in adults. In the case of infants, especially, giving them extra is certainly not better for them. Vitamin A levels above ten times the daily requirement for anyone can result in toxicity. Vitamin A should not be taken continually in amounts greater than the RDA for your age and sex.

The fortification of skim milk and nonfat dried milk with vitamin A to replace that removed with the cream is required by federal regulation. The same regulation requires the addition of vitamin A to margarine at the same level as it occurs naturally in butter. The fortification of foods that are not natural vitamin A sources, especially ready-to-eat cereals, with 100 percent of adult vitamin A requirement is a questionable practice. There are foods you should eat to get vitamin A at more normal levels, and for the varied selection of minerals and fiber they provide as well. You will not get hypervitaminosis A from eating too many fruits and vegetables high in carotene.

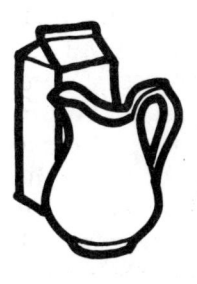

Vitamin D: The Sunshine Vitamin

Vitamin D has three functions all related to one another:

- It controls how and how much calcium and phosphorus are taken up from the digestive system.
- With one of the hormones, it plays a part in keeping the level of calcium and phosphorus in the blood constant.
- It controls how these minerals are transported to the bones, where they are deposited to mineralize the bones and give them strength.

Vitamin D plays a role in the formation and health of our bones, which depend also on adequate calcium and phosphorus intakes. The deficiency diseases caused by lack of vitamin D are discussed in the section on rickets and osteomalacia. One of the diseases, rickets, was once prevalent in smoggy and overcast northern climates and was referred to as the English disease. As far back as 1874 cod liver oil was mentioned, among other foods, as a cure for rickets. But it wasn't until 1918 that an English doctor proved the positive effect of cod liver oil, and it wasn't until 1925 that vitamin D, the antirachitic vitamin, was isolated. Since then rickets has been almost eliminated in countries where public health programs have seen that babies and children get vitamin D supplements during their growth years. Old-fashioned cod liver oil has been largely replaced by capsules of concentrated fish liver oils and synthetically made vitamin D.

Sources of Vitamin D

There are few food sources of vitamin D. A small amount is present in egg yolk and in the fat of milk; the richest natural source is fish liver oil, which is so concentrated that it is used as a supplement rather than a food. Sunshine is our main source of vitamin D, and has been down through history. One of the oils in your skin is a form of cholesterol which is converted to vitamin D when your skin is exposed to the ultraviolet rays of the sun. In this respect vitamin D is the only vitamin that is synthesized from another substance within the body tissues. For this reason the active form of vitamin D may in the future be classed as a hormone rather than a vitamin.

As a health measure, most of our milk supply is fortified to the level of a teenager's need per quart. Milk is a natural carrier for vitamin D because it contains fat to aid in its absorption. Milk is our best source of both calcium and phosphorus, with which vitamin D is functionally involved. The adult need for vitamin D is not known. A pint of fortified milk, the amount an adult needs for calcium, along with sunshine, will supply all the vitamin D that is probably needed.

How Much We Need

Vitamin D is vital for growth and bone structure, so the needs are greater in childhood, and during pregnancy and lactation. Vitamin D, like vitamin A, is measured in IU based on its curative effect. It is common for adults to think that since they are no longer growing, they need not bother about vitamin D. This is probably true in the summer for those living in the country or the suburbs, and all year for those living in sunny climates. But if you are a city worker, try to get some sunshine during your lunch hours. Very few people who travel by bus, subway, and automobiles get much sun on their way to and from work. Office buildings and schools with tinted windows also keep out the sun. It is better to try to get your vitamin D from the sun than from very highly fortified foods or vitamin concentrates.

We can get too much vitamin D. It is one of the four vitamins that we store in our bodies. It is stored in the liver and fatty tissue. This is an advantage, as the vitamin D made in our skin by exposure to the sun in summer provides some supply for the winter. But as in the case of vitamin A, if too much is taken, the body does not discard it, and toxic conditions can result. Intakes of from 1500 to 2000 IU can be harmful to babies and children. Intakes of five times those amounts cause calcium to be deposited in the wrong places, for example, in the soft tissues, instead of in the bones. A similar warning can be given to the elderly, who should not take high-level vitamin capsules without medical advice.

Because of the toxic effect of too much vitamin D, the fortification of foods other than milk with this vitamin is under review by the Food and Drug Administration (FDA). No health professional wishes to see a return of deficiency diseases, but as we learn more about the effects of overdoing a good thing, we are equally concerned about possible toxicity.

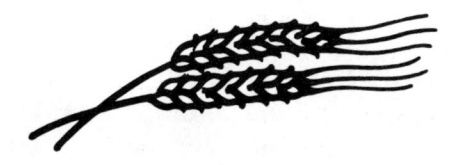

Vitamin E: An Enigma

Vitamin E has been described as a vitamin looking for a deficiency disease. Lack of vitamin E does not produce any clear-cut condition, but experiments with animals have shown that they need it for several functions. Research with human volunteers has not yet shown specific answers to the vitamin E enigma, but it has proven that we need vitamin E in the intricate function of body cells.

As with all vitamins, vitamin E functions in enzyme systems. In addition, vitamin E holds back oxidation where it should not occur. For example, it acts to protect certain cells and even nutrients on their way to meet the needs of the cells;

it protects vitamins A and C as they travel in the bloodstream; and it protects the red blood cells from the oxygen load they carry. Vitamin E is fat soluble and is involved with the oxidation of fats. The need for vitamin E goes up as the polyunsaturated fat content of the diet goes up. Those fats themselves usually contain a good amount of vitamin E, so the need is balanced.

Sources of Vitamin E

Vitamin E is present in many foods, so actual deficiencies of this vitamin are not seen in countries with an abundance of varied food. To study the effects of vitamin E, it has been necessary to have volunteers go on a diet lacking the vitamin. The best source of vitamin E is wheat germ. Unfortunately, wheat germ is removed from wheat for various reasons in the making of some cereals and flours. (Reasons for milling grain are discussed in chapter 11 under foods from grain.) But wheat germ as such is available; it is not removed from some cereals. Oils usually used for cooking and those in margarines are also excellent sources, as are egg yolk, liver, and green leafy vegetables.

Vitamin E is lost in food processing by removal, as with cereals. Since it is also lost in the freezing of fried foods and vegetables, it's not a good idea to rely too heavily on such prepared dinners for vitamin E.

How Much We Need

The National Academy of Sciences recognized vitamin E as an essential nutrient in 1968. The first mention of it occurred in 1922. In 1936 the "active" factor in vitamin E extracts was isolated in pure form and named alpha-tocopherol. It is measured in IU in the manner of fat-soluble vitamins A and D, but the IU of vitamin E is based on an amount of the pure vitamin. One IU of vitamin E is the activity of 1 milligram of alpha-tocopherol acetate.

In 1968, on the basis of research findings, recommended allowances were set at 30 IU for men and 25 IU for women. On the basis of research done between 1968 and 1973 the amounts were lowered in 1974 to 15 IU for men and 12 IU for women. The amount for babies (4 IU) is higher in relation to body weight because they are born with no stored supply. Children require a gradual increase to the adult level from ages 11 to 12.

During this time their overall increase in food intake covers their needs. (See the RDA table on page 96.) It has been observed that the more polyunsaturated fat in the food you eat, the more vitamin E you need. On the other hand, selenium, one of the trace minerals, can take the place of vitamin E in some way and reduce your need. This fact again illustrates the interrelationship of nutrients as they work in balance with one another.

Can we get too much? Vitamin E, like the other fat-soluble vitamins, is stored in your body. It is present in all cells, especially in certain glands, but is stored in the fatty tissue. While no toxic effects of taking large amounts of vitamin E have been documented in humans, they have been documented in animals. Signs of overdosage may yet appear since this vitamin has been promoted as a cure-all for humans.

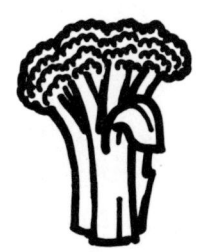

Vitamin K

Vitamin K is the catalyst for the formation of the factors that make our blood clot—when we are injured by a cut, for example. The last of the fat-soluble vitamins to be discovered (1935), it was made in pure form in 1939.

We don't have to be too concerned about intake or lack of vitamin K, because in addition to what we get in food we have friendly bacteria in the digestive tract that manufacture it. Taking antibiotic drugs can put these out of action and thus have a short-term effect on the supply. Food sources are green leafy vegetables, egg yolk, and liver. We store only a small amount of vitamin K. No RDA has been determined. There are no known dietary deficiencies, except in disease conditions in which vitamin K is included in the total treatment. A lack can occur in persons taking anticoagulants and mineral oil, which upsets the absorption from the digestive tract. Large amounts of synthetic vitamin K are toxic. The FDA has prohibited its use in vitamin supplements.

WATER SOLUBLE VITAMINS

B-Complex

The health and proper functioning of millions of our body cells depend on the vitamins of the B-complex. The cells depend for their sources of energy and for the materials for repair and replacement on reactions in which the B vitamins play coenzyme roles. They make the nutrients available for the cells' purposes and life. They are coenzymes in the metabolism of carbohydrate, fats, and protein—the three energy-giving nutrients—and in the synthesis of protein.

The busy metabolic processes of the body can be compared with the dance ensemble numbers in the great movie musicals of the thirties. The dancers link in twos, fours, eights, or all together, and then whirl around creating patterns and designs on the set. If even one dancer is missing, the effect is spoiled. Of the almost 50 known nutrients, 9 are B-vitamins, so when any one of them is missing, metabolic functions are interrupted or come to a halt. Fortunately, the B-vitamins are available in a wide selection of foods, but unfortunately, they are water soluble and sensitive to heat and light. Thus, they are easily lost in discarded cooking water, high-heat cooking, and food processing for long shelf life.

The intricate functions of the B-vitamins have been traced by research nutritionists using radioactive vitamins fed to animals and human volunteers. While this method has shown some fascinating processes of cell life, other functions still elude the nutrition researchers. Today, we know the following about the B-vitamins:

- There are at least nine of them.
- A daily supply is vital. You store very little if any of them in your tissues. Some are made by friendly bacteria in your digestive tract.
- Since other substances can make up for deficiencies of some of the B-vitamins, these deficiencies may not show up right away.
- Stress such as an illness can bring on deficiencies if your diet has had only marginal amounts of B-vitamins.

The three classic B-vitamin deficiencies are beriberi, brought on by a lack of thiamin; pellagra, caused by a lack of niacin; and anemias, caused by lacks of vitamin B_{12} or folacin.

In cases of beriberi and pellagra, the diet is usually deficient in other B-vitamins and other nutrients. Anemias caused by vitamin B_{12} or folacin deficiencies can be due to lack of only the one nutrient.

Thiamin: Vitamin B_1

Fifty percent of our body thiamin is in our muscles. Thiamin combines with phosphorus in enzymes and coenzymes that pass oxygen along to the tissues. Each step in the conversion of glucose to energy, carbon dioxide, and water takes place in this way. If this process is stopped at any stage, the compounds at that stage build up until they have a toxic effect that produces deficiency symptoms. For example, one of the most vital needs for thiamin is to bring about the change of pyruvic acid to lactic acid in a working muscle. The working muscle needs energy. If the thiamin coenzyme isn't there with its quota of oxygen to complete the steps of the energy cycle, the muscle goes into cramp as the energy supply stops and the pyruvic acid builds up. Nerves deprived of energy cannot transmit proper impulses to muscles. Thiamin is also a coenzyme in the release of energy from fats and from protein when it is used for energy. Without thiamin, the cells do not get energy from any one of our three energy sources.

In extreme and long-term deficiencies, beriberi results (discussed below). In marginal deficiencies, you will benefit noticeably from eating foods that supply your thiamin need. Adequate thiamin promotes good appetite and a properly functioning digestive system. This results in better growth in the growing years. Adequate thiamin will correct poor stamina, increase the ability to concentrate, and reduce irritability. It will also help in recovery from fatigue and prevent muscle cramp, various pains, and headaches.

We need thiamin every day. Our tissues take up only what they need and excrete any extra. To check your diet to see if you are getting enough, compare your daily food intake with that recommended in The Backbone of Good Nutrition, page 206. If you are eating a balanced diet and have any of the above conditions, they are probably not related to thiamin, and you should see a doctor.

Thiamin Deficiency: Beriberi

Thiamin deficiency, or beriberi, is the second most prevalent deficiency disease in today's world. Thiamin is needed to complete the steps of the change of glucose to energy for all nerves, all muscles, and the brain. When this process is stopped because the thiamin coenzyme is missing, the results are devastating. First the fingers are not able to feel, and eventually death results from paralysis and the inability of the heart muscle to beat.

Beriberi is seen in countries where the major source of calories in the diet is refined, or polished, rice. The outer coating of the natural wheat-colored grain is removed by polishing to make the rice white. Thiamin is in the brown coating of all grains. Another method of removing the brown coating is by steaming the rice. This dissolves the thiamin, and other B-vitamins which are absorbed into the remaining white grain. Thus parboiled rice has a higher vitamin content than polished rice. Beriberi was first discovered as a nutritional deficiency disease (as was scurvy) by a navy medical officer named Takaki who was puzzled by the death rate of his sailors. In 1878 Takaki increased the meat allowance and added milk to the sailors' rations. The crews stayed healthy, and the death rate dropped to zero.

In 1897 a Dutch scientist working in Java discovered that feeding chickens rice bran cured them of an odd nerve disease similar to beriberi. In 1901 another Dutch doctor, also in Java, fed rice bran to beriberi patients with curative results. Rice bran and wheat bran extracts are sold in health food stores on the basis of this old research. It is doubtful that they are tested for vitamin value as carefully as synthetically made B-vitamins.

In 1911 a factor was isolated from rice-bran extract by Dr. Funk who called it beriberi *vitamine*. In 1915 Dr. McCollum, who had named fat-soluble vitamin A, called a growth factor he was working on *water-soluble B*. It too cured the nerve disease. Continued work showed water-soluble B to be two vitamins. In 1925 they were called B_1 for the nerve factor and B_2 for the special growth factor. In 1926, the beriberi curative, B_1, was isolated in crystalline form and called thiamine (now thiamin). Ten years later it was made synthetically. Although people suffering from beriberi probably have other nutritional deficiencies, it was apparent after thiamin was isolated that the devastating effects of beriberi—damage to the tissues, destruction of nerves and muscles, and eventual paralysis—was really caused by the lack of thiamin.

Beriberi is still prevalent in the Orient and the islands of the

Pacific, where it is closely related to the people's food habits in that polished rice is still a large part of their diet. Some enrichment of rice is accomplished, but not in every locality. Most of the people do a lot of hard manual work, which demands high energy, which increases thiamin need. They eat raw fish, which contains a thiamin-destroying enzyme (thiaminase), and often have intestinal diseases that affect absorption of all nutrients.

Ever since thiamin was produced in crystalline form, it has been measured in milligrams. Because thiamin is essential for the release of energy from carbohydrates, the need for thiamin depends on the carbohydrate content of your diet. In general, it depends on the total energy content of the diet. Half a milligram for every 1000 calories has been set as the recommended allowance. For the needs of all ages and calorie levels, see the table of RDAs on page 97.

In present-day society, the persons most likely to be getting insufficient thiamin daily are alcoholics or heavy users of alcohol. Alcoholics often eat very poorly and are usually deficient in all B-vitamins and many nutrients. In addition, alcohol must be metabolized; it is a vitamin-free source of energy (almost as high as fat) and therefore increases the need for thiamin for anyone who has several drinks every day.

Since no food is exceptionally high in thiamin, we must eat a selection of foods to get our daily supply. Whole grains are good sources, but much thiamin is lost in milling and processing. This is why breads and cereals are enriched. Liver and organ meats are good sources, and pork is the best of muscle meats. Dried beans are a good source, as are leafy vegetables and milk if enough is consumed. Thiamin is lost when foods are cooked in water or at high temperature.

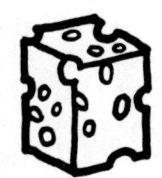

Riboflavin

When solutions containing the vitamin water-soluble B were heated, it was found to be two vitamins, B_1 and B_2. Heating destroyed water-soluble B's ability to cure the nerve condition eventually known as thiamin deficiency, but it did not seem to affect the ability to promote growth. The heat-resistant growth factor was called B_2. Much research on the B-vitamins was going on at that time and similar growth-promoting substances were found in liver, milk, eggs, and yeast, as well as in the bran coats of rice and wheat. These substances were called *flavins*. In 1932 a yellow enzyme necessary for cell life was extracted from yeast, and before long the growth-promoting flavins were identified as being the same as this enzyme. In 1935 they were given the common name of *riboflavin*. Later that year, riboflavin was synthesized.

Riboflavin is a component of enzymes that make hydrogen available for the work of your body cells, as thiamin does oxygen. Some are needed in the energy cycle to assist in the steps of energy release from both carbohydrates and fat. One of the end products of energy metabolism is water in which hydrogen is linked to oxygen.

Other riboflavin coenzymes are needed in your body's use of amino acids. Since amino acids are units for building protein, riboflavin assists in the process of growth and in the repair and replacement of cells.

How Much Riboflavin We Need

Ariboflavinosis is the name given to a deficiency of riboflavin. The symptoms of this disease are less severe than those of beriberi, partly because your body hangs on to its riboflavin supply very tightly when your diet is lacking in it. The health of many tissues is affected by a long-term lack of riboflavin. For example: skin is affected with seborrheic dermatitis, appearing especially around the nose; lips crack at the corners of the mouth, and there may be a change in the appearance of the tongue; eyes tire, are oversensitive to light, itch, feel as though they have sand in them, and vision is blurred; prolonged riboflavin deficiency may possibly be related to cataracts; and growth is slowed or stopped in children.

Riboflavin was made in crystal form soon after it was isolated as a vitamin. It is measured in milligrams. In 1968 the requirement was based on body size because riboflavin plays a role in the use of amino acids. In 1974 the recommended allowances were based on energy intake. There is little difference calculated either way; the energy calculation is simpler.

We need riboflavin every day. We store a small amount in our tissues. But when your tissues have taken up all the riboflavin they can, any excess is excreted. (See the table of RDAs, page 97, for all ages, especially for children and pregnant women, since riboflavin is a growth factor.) Riboflavin is present in many foods. Milk and cheese are our best sources. Liver, eggs, and yeast are also rich sources. Legumes, whole grain and enriched cereals, and leafy green vegetables, are good sources. As in the case of vegetables containing carotene, green vegetables containing riboflavin are also digested better when they are cooked. Riboflavin is not affected by heat in cooking, but it is soluble so can be lost in the cooking water.

Riboflavin deficiency is a problem in countries where people have a poor food supply. Recent studies show that there is some evidence of riboflavin deficiency in our own population, because of poor choice of foods and decreased milk consumption.

Niacin

Niacin is a component of two enzymes—coenzyme I and coenzyme II. They work in a manner similar to thiamin and riboflavin in changing glucose to energy. They are also needed to change glucose to glycogen, which is our only storage of carbohydrate. And they have a role in the synthesis of fat and cholesterol.

Pellagra: Niacin Deficiency Disease

Just as beriberi is a disease prevalent where the major food is polished rice, pellagra is a deficiency disease prevalent where the major food is corn. Pellagra was a major debilitating disease in the southern United States at the turn of this century. The disease is characterized by dermatitis, which appears on exposed skin and looks like sunburn; diarrhea or acute disturbance of the digestive system; dementia, which appears as confusion, irritability, delirium, and in some cases insanity.

The diet of the people of the southern states where pellagra was rampant was based on cornmeal, meat, and molasses. In 1915 a public health official, Dr. Goldberger, decided to find out if pellagra was a deficiency disease. He was convinced that there was something similar to B_1 and B_2 missing from the diet of persons with pellagra. In 1926 he found it in yeast and called it the pellagra-preventive (P-P) factor. In 1937 this factor was identified as being the same as nicotinic acid, which cured a similar deficiency condition in dogs. Nicotinic acid was given to pellagra patients that same year, and by 1945 pellagra had all but disappeared in the south. The name of the new vitamin was changed to niacin in 1971.

In most deficiency diseases, there is usually more than one nutrient lacking. In many cases, nutrients are needed together; while in others a nutrient can take the place of another. The latter is the case with niacin, which can be made in your body from the essential amino acid, tryptophan. This explains why an increase of even a small amount of high-quality protein in the diet can relieve symptoms of pellagra. It also explains why a diet of corn, which lacks tryptophan, is related to the incidence of pellagra. Soaking corn in lime makes its niacin more available. Mexicans have always done this before grinding corn to make tortillas, and because their diet is also high in legumes, which supply tryptophan, pellagra has never been a health problem in Mexico.

How Much Niacin We Need

Niacin, like thiamin and riboflavin, is measured in milligrams; 60 milligrams of tryptophan in your food counts as 1 milligram of niacin. Niacin is related to energy release, so the requirement is based on calorie level, with a minimum of 13 milligrams daily. (See RDA table, page 97.)

Sources of Niacin

Liver and yeast are the most concentrated sources of niacin. Meats, poultry, fish, and legumes are the best commonly eaten food sources, and they also supply tryptophan. Whole wheat, enriched cereals and leafy vegetables make a good contribution of both niacin and tryptophan.

If you have a healthy digestive system, you may manufacture some niacin which adds to your food supply. Taking sulpha drugs and antibiotics interrupts this synthesis.

Vitamin B_6

Vitamin B_6 was first identified in 1934. It was found to be necessary in experimental animals for growth and for the prevention of a skin disorder similar to that of deficiencies of the B-group. Since 1938, when B_6 was first made as pure crystals and called pyridoxine, two other forms of it have been discovered.

Vitamin B_6, usually joined with phosphorus, acts as a cofactor for a great number of enzymes, all of them involved with the use of the amino acids in the body. The enzyme functions include the following:

- Changing nonessential amino acids from one into another
- Changing tryptophan into niacin
- Making antibodies to fight infections
- Making hormones
- Forming the protein base for red blood cells
- Changing the amino acids so they can be used for energy when necessary.

Vitamin B_6 plays a part in changing glycogen to glucose, and it may be involved in changes in the fatty acids. The long list of complex reactions attributed to vitamin B_6 continues as research probes deeper into this intriguing vitamin.

There has never been a definitive deficiency disease condition of this vitamin in adults. The first knowledge we had of a need for the vitamin came when infants were fed a formula in which the B_6 had been destroyed by processing. They became very ill to the point of having convulsions. Adults who have gone on an experimental diet have shown that the lack of pyridoxine affects protein metabolism and all body functions that depend on protein. Experiments also showed that when the protein of the diet was increased, the B_6 need also increased. Other symptoms were similar to those resulting from a lack of riboflavin and niacin.

How Much We Need

As a result of the research on vitamin B_6 the Food and Nutrition Board in 1968 established a recommended allowance measured in milligrams. The requirement was based on the amount required to cure the symptoms caused by experimental deficiency. Your need increases when your diet is very high in protein, during pregnancy, if you are elderly, or if you are taking certain medications, including birth control pills and hormones. Alcoholics show B_6 deficiency symptoms along with deficiencies of the other B-vitamins. See the RDA table on page 97 for needs for all ages.

Sources of Vitamin B_6

The best sources of vitamin B_6 are those containing the other B-vitamins—liver, meat, whole grain cereals, legumes, and leafy vegetables. Most of the vitamin B_6 is lost when wheat is made into white flour. Processing of other foods also has a destructive effect on the vitamin. As people eat more and more precooked, preheated foods, vitamin B_6 deficiency could become a clinical reality.

Pantothenic Acid

Pantothenic acid, which is present in all living cells, was first identified in 1933 as another growth factor in the B-complex. Its name derives from a Greek word *panthos,* meaning "everywhere." Pantothenic acid was made in crystalline form in 1940. It is a component of coenzyme A, one of the most important enzymes in our whole life process. Coenzyme A is a master control enzyme. Despite this vital position, no deficiency of pantothenic acid has ever been seen in man, possibly because there is evidence we manufacture it in the digestive tract if we are in good health. So far as is known, pantothenic acid works with the other B-vitamins (riboflavin, niacin, pyridoxine, and biotin) and with the minerals phosphorus, sulphur, manganese, and magnesium.

Our need for pantothenic acid has not been quantitatively determined; consequently, there is no recommended dietary allowance. A suggested intake of 5 to 10 milligrams has been made, with the larger amount suggested for pregnant and lactating women.

Sources of Pantothenic Acid

Pantothenic acid is present in all naturally occurring foods. Sources with the highest concentration follow the pattern of the other B-vitamins, with liver, eggs, and wheat germ at the top. All meats, milk, legumes, peanuts, whole grains, and vegetables are good sources. Pantothenic acid is also found in fruits, something not true of the others of the B group except for folacin. There is not much loss of pantothenic acid in ordinary cooking, although there is some evidence of considerable losses in the processing of some foods. In milling grain, 50 percent of the pantothenic acid is lost and not replaced by enrichment. Freezing and canning also affect pantothenic acid. It is an optional vitamin included in nutrition labeling regulations. Some part of your daily intake must be raw or freshly cooked food, as we mentioned in our discussion of vitamin B_6. New vitamin deficiency conditions might appear with the increased use of processed foods.

Folacin

Because each of the B-vitamins is necessary for the utilization of other nutrients, any deficiency affects growth. Even after seven vitamins of the B-group had been isolated, unidentified growth factors remained. In 1941 one of these was isolated from spinach leaves and called folic acid (from the word *foliage*). In 1946 it was made in crystalline form. Folic acid was found to exist in other chemical variations, and the term *folacin* was adopted for the group. Its chemical name is *pteroylglutamic acid*.

Folacin is one of the most important of all the vitamins. On the other hand, it could be the vitamin more people in the world get in marginal amounts than any of the others we know. Folacin is the essential coenzyme in the renewal of our body cells. For example, the cells of the healthy digestive tract are renewed every three days. How folacin brings about this function of the cells is not yet precisely or fully understood. We do know that it synthesizes some amino acids in the process and that it uses vitamin B_6 to do so. We also know that folacin, as it travels in the blood to the cells, is protected from oxidation by vitamin C. The more we learn about each nutrient, the more we learn about how they depend on each other.

Folacin Deficiency

A lack of folacin affects the health and normal functioning of your digestive tract. A prolonged deficiency can result in diarrhea and poor absorption of nutrients from food. And conversely, conditions of the digestive tract, such as prolonged diarrhea or the presence of intestinal parasites, can bring about folacin deficiency. Folacin's most important activity is producing new red blood cells. Red blood cells have a life of about 30 days, and folacin is the enzyme that makes sure new cells are completely finished before being released to the blood stream. When folacin is lacking, the red cells are not properly formed and do not have their full amount of hemoglobin. This condition, called macrocytic anemia, is sometimes seen in women in their last months of pregnancy and during the period of breast-feeding. It is also seen in alcoholics and elderly persons living on poor diets.

How Much Folacin We Need

Folacin is measured in micrograms because compared to the other vitamins our needs for folacin are very small. Since a deficiency of folacin due to dietary errors is now recognized apart from other B-vitamin deficiencies, an RDA for adults of 400 micrograms was established in 1974. The amount is based on what is needed to cure macrocytic anemia (50 micrograms a day), plus a margin for safety. The need is greater during infancy, pregnancy, and breast-feeding.

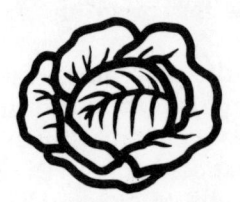

Sources of Folacin

We produce a fair amount of folacin in our digestive tract if we are healthy, but even so, we need some additional folacin from food. The best foods are the usual vitamin B sources—liver, yeast, legumes, nuts, and whole grains. Green leafy vegetables are also good sources, and oranges, surprisingly, have a high folacin content. Taking folic acid in vitamin capsules can hide the symptoms of pernicious anemia (see vitamin B_{12}, below), so the FDA has set a limit on the amount which can be put in a capsule. Many such capsules do not contain any folacin.

Vitamin B_{12}

Vitamin B_{12} was the last of the B-complex to be isolated. It took until 1948, and soon after, it was made in crystalline form from liver extract. Its chemical name is *cyanocobalamin,* as it has cobalt in its molecular structure. The discovery of vitamin B_{12} not only ended the search for all of the B-vitamins but it ended the search for the cause and treatment of pernicious anemia. Vitamin B_{12} is essential for the normal functioning of all the cells of your body, particularly the cells of your bone marrow (where blood is made) and of your nervous system and digestive tract. It plays a role in the metabolism of carbohydrate, fat, and protein—the three major energy nutrients—not for energy, but for rebuilding and constant replacement of all your body cells.

Control of Pernicious Anemia

Pernicious anemia was a fatal disease until 1926. In that year, two Boston doctors found that patients who ate a large amount of liver every day survived. This presented a clue that the disease might be a deficiency disease, and research proceeded in that direction. In pernicious anemia, as in folacin deficiency, red blood cells are not completely formed; there is also eventual degeneration of the spinal cord.

It was found that pernicious anemia was caused not by a lack of a food factor, but by lack of a factor in the digestive system that made it possible for the food factor to be absorbed through the intestinal walls into the blood stream. The liver factor was named the "extrinsic factor", and the digestive factor, produced in the stomach, the "intrinsic factor." Concentrated liver extracts were developed for pernicious anemia patients to relieve them of the need to eat liver every day. The liver factor became known as the "anti-pernicious anemia factor." Finally, in 1948 it was isolated in crystalline form and called vitamin B_{12}.

Today, pernicious anemia patients get once-a-month injections of vitamin B_{12} to keep them well. The anemia, which seems to be hereditary, is not actually cured but is kept under control.

Vitamin B_{12} deficiency has been seen in persons other than those with inherent pernicious anemia when there was a lack of the vitamin in their diet. Vitamin B_{12} is present only in foods of animal origin. Vegetarians who eat no milk or eggs as well as no meat can develop a deficiency. They do not develop pernicious anemia, or even anemia, but have symptoms similar to those caused by a lack of other B-vitamins—for example sore mouth and tongue, loss of weight, and lack of energy and vitality. But their nerves are affected to the degree of partial paralysis like the early nerve changes in pernicious anemia.

Any condition that affects the absorption of nutrients from the digestive tract can also cause a deficiency of vitamin B_{12}, for example, the disease tropical sprue, the presence of intestinal parasites, and even stomach surgery.

How Much We Need

Like folacin, vitamin B_{12} is measured in micrograms, since our needs are small. In 1968 vitamin B_{12} was included for the first time in the RDAs because deficiency conditions had been seen in persons eating no foods of animal origin. See the table on page 97 for needs for all ages.

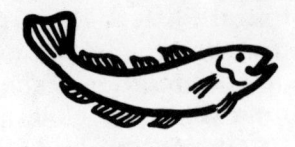

Sources of Vitamin B_{12}

Vitamin B_{12} is found only in foods of animal origin. Liver, of course, is an exceptional source. Milk, eggs, meat, fish and poultry provide us with vitamin B_{12}. Plants, including yeast, that are good sources of the other B-vitamins, provide no B_{12}. Vitamin B_{12} is destroyed by heat so some is lost in cooking, and especially if foods are processed at high temperatures.

Biotin

Biotin is another vitamin of the B-complex needed for proper growth. A deficiency of it results in lack of energy and causes skin changes and digestive disturbances similar to those seen in deficiency states of some others of the B-group. Like the others, it is a coenzyme and works with pantothenic acid in coenzyme A. It is needed for the synthesis of fatty acids, the release of energy from glucose, and in making some of the amino acids.

As with pantothenic acid, no deficiency has been seen in man except experimentally. Our dietary need for it has not yet been determined because a great amount of the biotin we need is made for us by bacteria in our digestive tract. Food sources are liver, egg yolk, legumes, and nuts. Raw egg white prevents biotin from being absorbed, and antibiotics affect its synthesis.

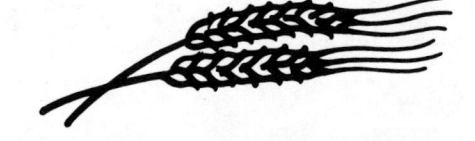

Choline

From research with animals, it has been learned that choline is a B-vitamin. No deficiency of it has been seen in people. The food need for it has not been established. You make choline in your digestive tract and it also occurs widely in food. Food sources of choline are egg yolk, liver, whole grains, legumes, milk, and meats.

From animal studies, choline has been shown to be present in all living cells. It is part of the compound needed to transmit nerve messages to the brain. It has a role in transporting fats and in their use by the body. Choline seems to prevent fat from building up in the liver in abnormal amounts; but it does not cure this condition if caused by disease or alcoholism.

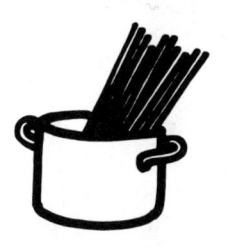

Some Things to Remember About the B-Vitamins

A lack of any one of the B-vitamins produces similar symptoms to the lack of another. Since loss of appetite, anemia, and headache can have other physiological causes, your doctor should determine, sometimes by simple blood tests, if you have a deficiency of the B-vitamins or some other problem. Taking high doses of the B-vitamins on your own can mask other conditions.

You do not store (or store very little of) the B-vitamins. If you are in good health, taking more than you need from high-potency capsules is not beneficial because the surplus vitamins are excreted. The absorption and in many cases the production of the B-vitamins is affected by medication, especially antibiotics and sulpha drugs. Do not take these on your own. The effect of taking hormones on the need for some of the B-vitamins is under study.

Much B-complex research was done on extracts of foods that contained the highest concentration of the factors under study. Yeast, liver, and the bran from rice and wheat were chief among them. The specific vitamins have long since been identified. Our traditional foods have been analysed and we now know which are sources of the B-vitamins. Health food stores sell the sources based on early research. There are no better sources of the B-vitamins than milk, meats, and fresh vegetables. If on your doctor's advice you need more of any of the B-vitamins than your diet supplies, you will be more sure of getting them from properly assayed sources checked by the FDA.

You can get all you need of the B-vitamins from a diet of fresh or freshly prepared traditional foods.

Ascorbic Acid: Vitamin C

Nutritionists agree in general on the function and need for the various nutrients, but they are not in total agreement on the role and the amount of vitamin C needed, particularly in relation to how it defends the body against infection.

Vitamin C, or ascorbic acid, has several functions on which nutritionists do agree. How vitamin C works in each of these vital functions is still being studied.

The most important function of vitamin C is in the formation of collagen, the protein substance of the connective tissue. Collagen is the material that holds the body cells (and us) together. Because of this function, vitamin C plays a role in the healing of burns and wounds from accidents or surgery. Vitamin C keeps the walls of the blood vessels strong, including those of the smallest capillaries. It helps in absorbing iron from the digestive system and in the formation of hemoglobin, the iron compound in the red blood cells. It plays a part in the use of amino acids and is needed for the synthesis of some hormones. It is important in the formation of substances that transmit nerve messages, and it protects vitamins A and E and the essential fatty acids from oxidation. It also helps your body fight infections.

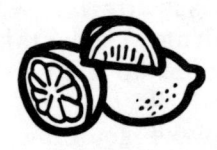

Vitamin C Deficiency

Scurvy is a degenerative disease that has been known since early Egyptian times. It appears as such in historical writings until it was discovered in the late eighteenth century that certain foods were protective. Ancient Greek soldiers on short rations developed gum disorders and painful legs. Many of the

Crusaders died from scurvy. People held captive in cities under siege fell to the disease. In times of crop failure and famine, scurvy reaped its toll. Sailors on long voyages developed scurvy, and usually more than half of the crews died from it.

A Scottish doctor in the British navy was so appalled by the loss of sailors that he set out to find the cause. He experimented by adding different foods to the rations of a group of sailors. The sailors who received lemon juice stayed healthy and showed no signs of scurvy. This was in 1753. When Captain Cook made his trip around the world from 1772 to 1775, he took on fresh fruits and vegetables at every port with the result none of his crew died of scurvy. The substance in lemon juice that prevented scurvy was first called *antiscorbutin*. Then it was called vitamin C in the alphabetic naming of the vitamins. It was finally isolated in crystalline form in 1932, and the following year it was named ascorbic acid, a shortened version of its original name.

Scurvy is rarely seen today, but the symptoms of scurvy point to the many areas of the body that are affected by vitamin C deficiency. Outright scurvy causes degeneration of the blood vessel walls, muscles, bones, teeth, gums, and skin. The same tissues are affected by a marginal lack of vitamin C. Your gums become sore and bleed easily. You bruise easily because capillaries are weakened. You may have pains in your joints. A minor deficiency will also make you less resistant to infection. Children who have vitamin C deficiency do not grow properly, and they also suffer pains in the bones and joints. The "growing pains" of the last century were probably mild scurvy, as they usually occurred in spring after a winter diet lacking fresh fruits and vegetables. Babies and children who have vitamin C deficiency are irritable, restless, and don't like to be touched.

How Much We Need

There is much controversy over the amount of vitamin C you need—not so much as how much is your daily requirement, but whether extra amounts will protect you from infection, especially the common cold.

Vitamin C (ascorbic acid) has been measured in milligrams ever since it was made in the pure form. The amount you need to protect you from symptoms of scurvy is quite small, about 10 milligrams. The recommended dietary allowance is set not too much above that amount in some countries. In the United States, it is set considerably higher, at 45 milligrams per day for adults. (See RDA table, page 97.)

There is some indication that stress and infection increase your need for vitamin C. We do not have a storage supply in our tissues, but all the tissues have a certain amount present. We have about 1500 milligrams in our bodies when healthy. Under stress and infection, this level can be lowered. Some nutritionists feel that vitamin C should be taken in increased amounts until the tissues are filled up or saturated again.

Once the tissues are saturated, however, they cannot take any more, so extra amounts above your needs are excreted. But once again, the body's ability to adapt to levels of nutrients shows up in persons who take large amounts of vitamin C constantly. Their bodies adapt to the high intake level, and then if they stop taking the vitamin, they can show the symptoms of mild deficiency. There seems to be no proven reason to take excessively high amounts of vitamin C. Indeed, there is more evidence that to do so could be harmful.

Exceptionally high levels of vitamin C have been suggested as a treatment for the common cold. This is a medicinal use of ascorbic acid apart from its role as a nutrient. Many question this use, and you should not use it this way unless your doctor advises you to do so for a short period. An intake of 1 gram taken for too long can show toxic effects.

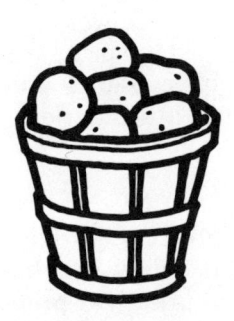

Sources of Vitamin C

The best sources of vitamin C are certain fruits—strawberries, oranges, grapefruit, melons, and papayas. The best vegetable sources are broccoli, tomatoes, cauliflower, green pepper, and leafy green vegetables whether they are cooked or raw. Freshly cooked turnips and baked potatoes are also good sources of the vitamin. Vitamin C is soluble in water and is affected by heat; thus some is lost in cooking.

Some vitamin C is lost in the processing of fruits and vegetables and in long-term storage. Ascorbic acid is added to many convenience foods as an antioxidant, which could supply us with small amounts. Vitamin C is added to some enriched cereals and to cereals labeled as dietary supplements.

Some fruits not common in this country have a high vitamin C value. Rose hips (seed pods) are one of these. They gained a place in the diet during World War II in Great Britain and Canada. Oranges do not grow in these countries, but roses thrive. During the war, rose hips were promoted as a source of vitamin C to avoid the necessity of importing citrus fruits. They are not particularly exciting to eat and are no match for a glass of fresh orange juice or half a papaya. Dried, as sold in health food stores, they are a dubious source of vitamin C.

6.

The Recommended Dietary Allowances and the U.S. Recommended Daily Allowances for Nutrition Labeling

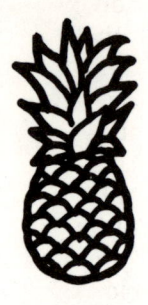

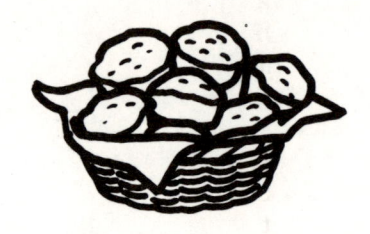

The Recommended Daily Dietary Allowances (RDAs) are the levels of intake of essential nutrients that are considered by the Food and Nutrition Board of the National Research Council to meet the known needs of healthy people. The Food and Nutrition Board, established in 1940, is an advisory board whose members are chosen from among leaders in food-related sciences. The Board promotes needed research and interprets work in nutrition in the interests of national health. Members are not paid for their services except for expenses.

The RDA table does not cover all nutrients that were described in the preceding chapters. Only seventeen of the almost 50 nutrients we require daily and the need for calories are given in the table that follows. At best, the RDA is a guide, and a diet made up of naturally occurring foods that contain the nutrients for which there are RDAs should keep us in good health. Keeping nutritional unknowns in mind, we should eat a varied diet. As new knowledge is acquired and accepted by the Board, RDAs are reviewed and revised every five years.

The RDA is a standard with a built-in safety level. It takes into account nutrients that may not be completely absorbed and allows extra above the estimated need. It also takes into account that the body stores some nutrients and conserves others when they are in short supply. The total is a liberal allowance and above the actual needs of many persons; it is not the absolute amount that you actually require. Many factors affect your individual requirements. The RDA is a guide for the population as a whole. It does not take into account the special needs of chronic or metabolic disorders or acute illnesses.

The RDA is a standard for a "reference person," a man or woman in good health, living a moderately active life. Your age, size, and activities are three things that determine your need for energy. The reference weight for men is 154 pounds; the height 5 feet 9 inches. The reference weight for women is 128 pounds; the height, 5 feet 5 inches. If you are under 21, you must remember that you also need an allowance for growth. If you look at the RDA table, you will see that the energy requirement for infants is given as a number times their weight. The needs through the growth period (to age 21) are calculated in a similar manner. (Nutrient and calorie intake in terms of food is covered in the last chapter of this book.)

The first edition of the RDA was established and printed in 1943 to provide "standards to serve as a goal for good nutrition." The eighth edition was published in 1974. Since the first edition, the RDA has become a standard in many areas. An early use was planning food supplies for the armed forces. It is now used in planning food supplies for other segments of the population, such as children whose lunches are provided by their schools. The RDA is used to interpret studies of food consumption, establish standards for public assistance programs, evaluate the adequacy of food supplies in meeting our national nutritional needs, develop educational programs, guide development of new products by the food industry, and set guidelines for nutrition labeling.

FOOD AND NUTRITION BOARD, NATIONAL ACADEMY OF SCIENCES–NATIONAL RESEARCH COUNCIL
RECOMMENDED DAILY DIETARY ALLOWANCES, REVISED 1974

	Age	Weight		Height		Energy	Protein	Fat-Soluble Vitamins		
								Vitamin A	Vitamin D	Vitamin E Activity
	(years)	(kg)	(lbs)	(cm)	(in)	(kcal)	(g)	(IU)	(IU)	(IU)
Infants	0.0–0.5	6	14	60	24	kg × 117	kg × 2.2	1,400	400	4
	0.5–1.0	9	20	71	28	kg × 108	kg × 2.0	2,000	400	5
Children	1–3	13	28	86	34	1,300	23	2,000	400	7
U.S. RDA (children)*							28	2,500	400	10
	4–6	20	44	110	44	1,800	30	2,500	400	9
	7–10	30	66	135	54	2,400	36	3,300	400	10
Males	11–14	44	97	158	63	2,800	44	5,000	400	12
	15–18	61	134	172	69	3,000	54	5,000	400	15
	19–22	67	147	172	69	3,000	54	5,000	400	15
	23–50	70	154	172	69	2,700	56	5,000		15
	51+	70	154	172	69	2,400	56	5,000		15
Females	11–14	44	97	155	62	2,400	44	4,000	400	12
	15–18	54	119	162	65	2,100	48	4,000	400	12
	19–22	58	128	162	65	2,100	46	4,000	400	12
	23–50	58	128	162	65	2,100	46	4,000		12
	51+	58	128	162	65	1,800	46	4,000		12
U.S. RDA (adults)**							45	5,000	400	30
Pregnant Females						+300	+30	5,000	400	15
Lactating Females						+500	+20	6,000	400	15

NOTE: The U.S. RDA (allowances) are based on the 7th edition of the RDA (1968).
The U.S. RDA for protein are 45 gms. for animal protein and 65 gms. for vegetable protein to make 100%.
* The U.S. RDA (children) is the standard for labeling baby and junior foods (ages 1 to 4).
** The U.S. RDA (adult) is the standard for labeling all food other than baby and junior foods.
The percentage of the U.S. RDA listed on package labels are percentages of these figures.
The U.S. RDA includes the following additional nutrients and allowances.
    Adult—copper 2 mg. biotin 0.3 mg. pantothenic acid 10 mg.
    Child—copper 1 mg. biotin 0.15 mg. pantothenic acid 5 mg.

Water-Soluble Vitamins							Minerals					
Ascorbic Acid (mg)	Folacin (mcg)	Niacin (mg)	Riboflavin (mg)	Thiamin (mg)	Vitamin B₆ (mg)	Vitamin B₁₂ (mcg)	Calcium (mg)	Phosphorus (mg)	Iodine (mcg)	Iron (mg)	Magnesium (mg)	Zinc (mg)
35	50	5	0.4	0.3	0.3	0.3	360	240	35	10	60	3
35	50	8	0.6	0.5	0.4	0.3	540	400	45	15	70	5
40	100	9	0.8	0.7	0.6	1.0	800	800	60	15	150	10
40	200	9	0.8	0.7	0.7	3.0	800	800	70	10	200	8
40	200	12	1.1	0.9	0.9	1.5	800	800	80	10	200	10
40	300	16	1.2	1.2	1.2	2.0	800	800	110	10	250	10
45	400	18	1.5	1.4	1.6	3.0	1,200	1,200	130	18	350	15
45	400	20	1.8	1.5	2.0	3.0	1,200	1,200	150	18	400	15
45	400	20	1.8	1.5	2.0	3.0	800	800	140	10	350	15
45	400	18	1.6	1.4	2.0	3.0	800	800	130	10	350	15
45	400	16	1.5	1.2	2.0	3.0	800	800	110	10	350	15
45	400	16	1.3	1.2	1.6	3.0	1,200	1,200	115	18	300	15
45	400	14	1.4	1.1	2.0	3.0	1,200	1,200	115	18	300	15
45	400	14	1.4	1.1	2.0	3.0	800	800	100	18	300	15
45	400	13	1.2	1.0	2.0	3.0	800	800	100	18	300	15
45	400	12	1.1	1.0	2.0	3.0	800	800	80	10	300	15
60	400	20	1.7	1.5	2.0	6.0	1,000	1,000	150	18	400	15
60	800	+2	+0.3	+0.3	2.5	4.0	1,200	1,200	125	18+	450	20
80	600	+4	+0.5	+0.3	2.5	4.0	1,200	1,200	150	18	450	25

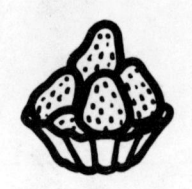

THE STANDARD FOR NUTRITIONAL LABELING: THE U.S. RDA

A regulation that encouraged food companies to give certain allowed nutritional information on the label came into effect in the United States in July, 1975. The standard on which this information is based is called the United States Recommended Daily Allowances or U.S. RDA. The U.S. Recommended *Daily* Allowances are a composite of the Recommended *Dietary* Allowances, and one should not be confused with the other.

The complete RDA gives 26 age-sex variables for each of the nutrients in the table. From these, the highest value has been chosen for each key nutrient, except calcium, from any age group above the age of four as the U.S. RDA standard for nutrition labeling. There is another U.S. RDA for the labeling of baby and junior food (ages 1 to 4). Thus, the U.S. RDAs represent the amounts of nutrients needed every day by healthy people, plus an excess of 30 to 50% to allow for individual variations. Many adults need only two-thirds to three-fourths of the U.S. RDA for several nutrients, and children only about half.

The U.S. RDA are based on the 1968 edition of the RDA. The legislative action was already in motion before the 1974 edition was published. The 1974 edition has some differences. The requirements for protein, vitamin C, vitamin E, and niacin were lowered; the requirement for riboflavin was increased; and a requirement for zinc was established.

In addition to the nutrients listed in the 1974 RDA, the U.S. RDA includes three nutrients for which no recommended allowances have yet been established. These are copper, pantothenic acid, and biotin. In the table on page 96 you can compare your needs depending on your age and sex with the U.S. RDA standard used for labels.

The U.S. RDA nutrient list established for labeling is divided into two groups. In one group are the nutrients that *must* be listed. The other group *may* be listed. The difference between the two groups is explained below in the section on what nutrition labeling tells you. If a food is naturally a very good source of a required nutrient, it is to the consumer's advantage to know. On the other hand, if a food manufacturer has added the optional nutrients to a product to make it appear superior to a natural food, this can mislead the consumer.

Many forces contributed to the passage of the labeling regulation.

- Consumer concern about the nutritional value of foods.
- Development of new products that replace naturally occurring, freshly cooked foods, possibly leading to lower nutrient intakes.
- Nutritionists' belief that information on highly refined foods that are subsequently highly fortified with nutrients should be made known to the consumer.
- Nutritionists' concern about the introduction of foods fabricated from highly purified ingredients and the disregard of the trace elements and remaining unknowns of nutrition.
- Greater health consciousness, especially in relation to food. At the same time, changed lifestyles make it difficult to estimate daily nutritional intake. For example, breakfasts on the run and meals eaten away from home are often unplanned food choices and consequently may add up to poor choices.

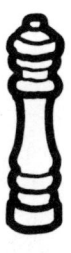

What Nutrition Labels Tell You

While labeling regulation is established on a voluntary basis, it is mandatory under two conditions.

1. If a nutrient has been added to a product either under "enrichment" regulation (see Chapter 10) or by "fortification," as the addition of vitamin D to milk, the label must provide nutritional information.

2. If any nutritional claim is made for the product on the label or in advertising, the product label must provide the mandatory nutritional information.

Food and Drug Administration (FDA) labeling regulations require that certain nutrition information be shown on a specific part of the label of cans and packages. The label must tell you:

- Number of servings in the container and size of the serving
- Caloric content of a serving
- Amount (in grams) of carbohydrate, fat, and protein in a serving
- Percentage of the U.S. RDA of protein, calcium, iron, vitamin A, vitamin C, thiamin, riboflavin, and niacin, in a serving
- Any added vitamin D, vitamin E, vitamin B_6, folacin, vitamin B_{12}, phosphorus, iodine, magnesium, zinc, copper, biotin, or pantothenic acid must be listed. They *may* be listed, if naturally present. If the product is made of 10 percent or more of fat or has more than 2 grams of fat in a serving, a description of the fat can be given. The cholesterol content may also be given. If the fats are described, the label must say:

"Information on fat and/or cholesterol content is provided for individuals who, on the advice of a physician, are modifying their total dietary intake of fat and/or cholesterol."

What the Labels Do Not Tell You

Nutrition labels do not tell you what the U.S. RDA percentage represents in terms of the actual amount of a nutrient. For labeling baby and junior foods there is a line (table, page 96) called the U.S. RDA for children ages 1 to 3. The amounts in that line are used as 100 percent of a child's need. Under the adult section is the U.S. RDA or amounts that are used as 100 percent of adult need. You can then compare your actual need for your age and sex, and also the needs of other members of your family, with the U.S. RDA.

For example, if you are a woman, your RDA for vitamin A is 4000 IU (International Units), as shown in the table. The percentage of vitamin A on the label of a food product is a percentage of the U.S. RDA which is 5000 IU. If the food contributes 20 percent of the U.S. RDA, it contains 1000 IU of vitamin A. Since 1000 IU is 25 percent (one quarter) of your RDA needs, the label understates the food's contribution of vitamin A to your needs.

A woman's needs are higher in pregnancy; for vitamin A they are the same as the U.S. RDA. If you are smaller than a reference woman, your needs are even less than the 4000 IU of the RDA. For this reason, and also because the RDAs are revised periodically, the food tables in the following chapters are based on the traditional weight system (grams, milligrams, and micrograms) rather than expressed as a percentage of the U.S. RDA.

The labels also do not tell you what percentage of the U.S. RDA makes a particular food a good source of a nutrient. Whether a food is a good source depends not only on how much is in a serving, but also on how many servings are usually eaten daily. If one serving of a food contributes 10 percent of the U.S. RDA, for example, you would have to have ten servings of it (or of an equivalent food) to reach 100 percent. A food source that has 10 percent of any one nutrient makes a good, though not exceptional, contribution to your total need. Nutrition labels do not tell you what the other foods are to make up the missing 90 percent. They tell you only about that particular food. Therefore, you must learn what foods are high sources of the many nutrients.

Labels are not required on fresh foods, some of which are the best sources of nutrients listed as well as those not listed.

Nutrition labels do not tell you how processed food differs from the fresh food, for example, how fresh potatoes differ from dried potato flakes. No information is given about nutrients that are not listed. It was originally assumed that if the important minerals calcium and iron were present in naturally occurring foods, together with vitamins A and C, thiamin, riboflavin, and niacin, then the food would also make a contribution of other nutrients, especially the trace minerals. But this is not the case with fabricated foods and highly processed and fortified foods. The nutrition information panel on the label does not tell you which nutrients have been added to the food, whether at "restored," "enriched," or "fortified" levels. But added nutrients have to be included in the ingredient listing.

What You Can Learn from Nutrition Labels

After considerable time and study, you may make better choices of foods from the 9,000 items in the supermarket, but you cannot learn nutrition while shopping. It is difficult to compare the nutritive values of different forms of the same food. For example, fresh green beans have no nutrition labeling, while canned green beans are in one aisle and frozen green beans are usually several aisles away. The nutritive value of the same food processed in the same way by different companies will not be significantly different. The best way to learn nutrition from labels is to save them and read them at home. You can then compare the values of different foods, especially of fruits and vegetables.

You can compare cereals more easily because they have all been processed to some degree; but you get great variation in nutritional value since this class of food comes under the enrichment laws and after the 1940s three of the B-vitamins were added to refined grain. In the last few years, cereal companies have added more and more vitamins and minerals as well. When a cereal contains nutrients in amounts that are 100 percent of the U.S. RDA, it must be labeled a "dietary supplement." The nutritional value of cereals is discussed further in Chapter 11.

Nutrition information labeling is based on the premise that the consumer has a right to know. Its success depends on you. Since providing such information on product labels is voluntary, some companies have chosen not to do so. This does not mean their product is necessarily inferior. These companies must put their name and address on the label, and you can write for nutrition information. Even if you inquire about only one nutrient, the company must send you all the information that would be required on a label. Consumers should remember the following points:

1. If a nutrient in a serving is less than 2 percent of the U.S. RDA, it cannot be mentioned. Sometimes when a food has under 2 percent of a nutrient in an average serving, the serving size is doubled in order that mention may be made of the nutrient—which of course gives an exaggerated amount of all the nutrients.

2. Although highly fortified foods appear to be higher in nutrients than traditional foods are, this is misleading; certain nutrients of the nearly 50 we know we need are present in traditional foods but not in processed fortified products.

3. No naturally occurring food is a rich source of all nutrients. Some are exceptional sources of only one. Such a natural food

makes a poor showing when labels are compared. For example, canned carrots are high in vitamin A, but have small percentages of the other nutrients.
4. Ingredients must be listed and information on additives (including nutritive additives) given on labels of food products. (See chapters on specific foods.)

7.
Milk and Milk Products

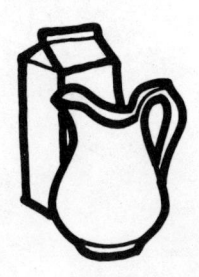

Milk is probably our most important single food. It is the first food we eat, and we never outgrow our need for it. Because of their exceptional qualities, milk and milk products constitute one of the major food groups of a balanced diet.

Milk is designed by nature as the perfect food for babies and young animals and is the only food they need for a matter of weeks. The milk of animals was recognized very early in history as having nutritional value for the weaned child and, when converted to other forms, for adults as well. Our centuries-old reliance on milk is illustrated in the history of many lands. The cow, as provider of milk, was used as part of a dowry, as a medium of exchange, as a measure of wealth—and in India, even became a sacred object. In today's economy, cow's milk continues to be a high-protein food produced at lower cost than the meat from steers or sheep. Milk cows are much more efficient in transforming feed into the protein of milk than steers and sheep are in the production of protein as meat. If future populations expand, this will be of greater significance. The many animals that have been providers of milk (goats, sheep, water buffalo, camel, reindeer, and yak) must continue to be looked to more than meat animals as sources of high-quality protein food.

MILK: A MULTINUTRIENT FOOD

Milk is 87 percent water; the other 13 percent contains more known nutrients—in amounts that are significant, well balanced, and easily assimilated—than any other single food. Pasteurized homogenized vitamin D milk, the standard milk in your grocery store, is fortified with vitamin D, but it has practically no vitamin C.

Building Materials for Bones and Teeth

Calcium and phosphorus, the two major minerals needed for building and maintaining bones and teeth, are present in milk in a favorable ratio. Milk is the principal food source of calcium in the North American diet. It is very difficult for you to get the amount of calcium you need daily from foods other than milk or cheese.

Vitamin D is the most important vitamin involved in the process of making well-formed and healthy bones and teeth. For this reason milk is fortified. The amount of vitamin D added is regulated by law and based on the RDAs. Milk so fortified is labeled "vitamin D milk."

Riboflavin

Riboflavin occurs naturally in milk, and milk is your best source of it. Milk supplies from 45 to 50 percent of your daily riboflavin requirement when you drink the amount required for your daily calcium needs. An adult should drink two 8-ounce glasses (1 pint) of milk daily, a teenager four glasses (1 quart), and growing children from two to four glasses, depending on their age. Riboflavin is quite stable when exposed to heat, but it is destroyed by light.

Protein

The proteins of milk have the highest biological value except for the protein of egg. The lactalbumin, lactoglobulin, and casein of milk contain all the essential amino acids in good proportion and are sources of additional lysine. The extra lysine of milk and milk products can supplement the amino acids of the protein of cereals, bread, and pasta and make a combined amino acid mixture that has as high a biological value as milk itself. Casein in the form of caseinate often appears in the ingredient listing of convenience foods. It is not an additive but a milk protein.

Vitamin A

Whole milk is a good source of vitamin A, which is in the fat of the milk. Vitamin A is removed with the fat when milk is skimmed, but vitamin A is restored to most skimmed-milk products. The level of restoration may be higher than the original and is set as a proportion of the RDA for vitamin A for adults. Milk so fortified is labeled "fortified with Vitamin A."

Fat (Cream)

The fat content of milk as it comes from the dairy cow is quite high. After cows were milked in days gone by, the milk was cooled and allowed to stand overnight. The fat or cream rose to the top, and the next day most of it was skimmed off to be made into butter. Because consumers in those days felt they were entitled to a certain amount of cream, laws were passed specifying how much cream or butterfat had to be left. These specifications are part of the milk standards (see page 108) and vary from state to state; 3.25 percent butterfat is the usual amount required.

The cream in liquid whole milk will rise naturally to the top, but most milk today is homogenized to prevent this. In homogenized milk the fat globules have been broken up by a mechanical process into minute droplets that remain distributed in the milk. Other than this, milk fats are unchanged by processing and contain their original enzymes and trace minerals. They also contain saturated, monounsaturated, and polyunsaturated fatty acids, including some of the essential fatty acid, linoleic acid. Milk fats are carriers of vitamins A and D and contain some cholesterol.

One advantage milk has over other animal protein foods is that the fat can be lowered and even completely removed with little expense, leaving a completely palatable product, skim milk. Thus, you can get milk's most valuable nutrients (calcium, riboflavin, protein, and vitamin A) and avoid fat by using skim milk fortified with vitamins A and D, usually labelled "Vitamin-A and -D Skim Milk."

Intolerance to Milk and Milk Sugar

Some of the energy value of milk comes from carbohydrate. The carbohydrate in milk is a sugar called lactose. The digestion of lactose requires the presence in the digestive tract of a specific enzyme, lactase. When you stop drinking milk, you may stop producing the enzyme. Some adults do not tolerate milk well, but they can usually tolerate acidulated milk, such as buttermilk, and other forms of milk, such as yogurt and cheese. It has been claimed that milk intolerance is a problem of ethnic groups that are not traditional milk drinkers after weaning. But most of these people can use milk in small quantities, and their children probably can develop greater tolerance if milk is included in their diets.

Other Nutrients

Milk is a vital source of vitamin B_{12} for people who do not eat meat, poultry, fish, or eggs for any reason. It also supplies significant but not major amounts of the B-vitamins—vitamin B_6, pantothenic acid, niacin, folacin, and some thiamin. The amount of iron in milk is not great, but it is in a form that you can absorb and use. As milk is the complete food for the infant, it contains other major elements—magnesium, sodium, potassium, chloride and sulphur—as well as the trace minerals zinc, copper, iodine, fluorine, manganese, molybdenum, cobalt, and chromium.

MILK LAWS AND STANDARDS FOR CONSUMER PROTECTION

After the French scientist Louis Pasteur discovered that bacteria caused certain diseases, it became possible to identify the bacteria that sometimes occur in raw milk—bacteria that cause tuberculosis, undulant fever, scarlet fever, and typhoid fever. Pasteurization makes milk completely safe by destroying these harmful bacteria. It is the process of heating every particle of milk (or milk product) to at least 145° F. (63° C) and holding it at or above this temperature for at least 30 minutes, or heating to at least 161° F. (71° C) and holding at or about this temperature for at least 15 seconds. The milk is cooled immediately following the heating. Pasteurization makes no significant change in flavor or food value other than decreasing milk's small amount of vitamin C.

The FDA established food standards to "promote honesty and fair dealing in the interest of the consumers." There are standards of identity and quality for most milk, cream, and cheese and for cheese products, ice cream, and related foods.

Labeling

All the ingredients in a product have to be listed by weight (not volume), in descending order, and the reason for any additives must be given. The law requires that if any nutrients have been added to the product the carton or package must provide nutritional information. Most pasteurized homogenized milk has added vitamin D, and most low-fat and skim milks have added vitamins A and D, so all these products must have nutritional information on the cartons.

Definitions and Standards of Some Other Milk Products

Raw milk has not been pasteurized. It is produced by inspected and certified dairy herds for special purposes.

Lowfat 2 percent milk is pasteurized fluid milk from which the butterfat has been removed to 2 percent. It must have vitamin A added, and may have vitamin D added.

Skim milk is pasteurized fluid milk from which the butterfat has been removed to 1 percent or less. It must have vitamin A added, and may have vitamin D added.

Protein fortified lowfat (2 percent) milk is pasteurized fluid milk from which the butterfat has been removed to 2 percent and to which has been added one or more of the following: nonfat dry milk, minerals, and vitamins. The composition of the product depends on the dairy that makes it; but the law requires that all ingredients be listed and nutritional information must be given.

Homogenized skim milk product is a pasteurized and homogenized blend of skim milk, whole milk, and nonfat dry milk solids with a total butterfat content of 1 percent, fortified with vitamins A and D.

The composition of protein-fortified lowfat milks and homogenized skim milk products varies within allowable limits from brand to brand. But because all have nutrients added, nutritional information will be on the carton. Fortifying them with vitamins A and D is nutritionally sound. Fortifying them with protein is unnecessary as milk is a naturally high protein food. However, when these products are the major source of protein in the diet, as they are for lacto-ovo vegetarians, they are economically and nutritionally sound.

Protein-fortified lowfat milk and homogenized skim milk products are also excellent for supplying the additional protein, calcium, and other nutrients demanded by pregnancy, without increasing fat intake. Children and teenagers also have high requirements for protein and calcium for growth, but they usually use up a lot of energy and need the linoleic acid in the fat of whole milk. If they do not have a high energy output, they should reduce their calorie intake from other sources, such as sweet snacks.

Both protein-fortified lowfat milk and homogenized skim milk products are good forms of milk for you if you are an adult of normal weight and have been advised to reduce your fat intake. But if you are trying to lose weight and are restricting your energy intake, then you should use regular skim milk because it is not as high in calories from both protein and milk sugar. Your diet will be better balanced if you choose foods within your calorie allotment that add nutrients not available in your skim milk allowance. The best choices would be fruits and vegetables, for their vitamin C, iron, and fiber.

Buttermilk is pasteurized skim milk to which a specially prepared culture and sometimes butter granules are added. It has a butterfat content of 1 percent or less.

Chocolate milk is whole milk with 1 percent cocoa or 1½ percent liquid chocolate, 5 percent sugar, and less than 1 percent stabilizers added. The mixture is then pasteurized.

Chocolate dairy drink is made of skim milk of about 2 percent butterfat and contains milk solids that are at least 90 percent of that of skim milk, plus cocoa, sugar, and stabilizers.

Evaporated milk is fluid whole milk which is pasteurized, concentrated by the removal of about half the water under vacuum, homogenized, fortified with 400 IU of vitamin D per pint, sealed in cans, and finally heat sterilized. It will keep without refrigeration for one year.

Sweetened condensed milk is fluid whole milk which is pasteurized, sweetened with a specific amount of sugar, concentrated by removing about half the water under vacuum, and then sealed in cans. Because it is from 40 to 50 percent sugar, it requires no heat treatment to prevent spoilage. It will keep without refrigeration for up to one year. This was the earliest method devised to preserve milk in a liquid state. It was used for feeding infants at the turn of the century, but we now know that its excessively high sugar content makes it most unsuitable for such purposes.

Instant nonfat dry milk fortified with vitamins A and D is fluid milk skimmed of all fat, then pasteurized, with part of the water removed by vacuum. It is then sprayed into a chamber of heated air, which evaporates the remaining water, and the solids fall to the bottom. The solids are then "instantized," or treated with steam and then redried, so that they will dissolve readily in water. The removal of the fat also removes the vitamins A and D, so the product has these vitamins added. When it is reconstituted according to package directions, its food value is the same as vitamin A and D fluid skim milk, and 8 ounces will contain 500 IU of vitamin A and 100 IU of vitamin D.

Yogurt is made from pasteurized homogenized whole or partially skim milk; yogurt is altered in flavor, acidity, and consistency by the addition of a culture, and sometimes milk solids as well. There is a proposed federal standard for the composition of yogurt. At present it can vary in fat content from about 1 to 7 percent, depending on the manufacturer.

Fruit-flavored yogurt is yogurt to which fruit has been added, usually in the form of preserves or jam. If nutritional information is given on the carton, the amount of carbohydrate listed will give an indication of the amount of preserves added. One cup of milk from which the yogurt is made will contain only 12 grams of carbohydrate. If the label states, for example, 25 grams of carbohydrate, then 13 grams are from preserves.

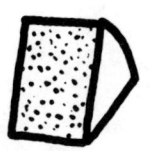

CHEESE AND CHEESE PRODUCTS

Cheese is the fresh or matured product obtained by draining after the coagulation of milk, cream, skimmed or partly skimmed milk, buttermilk, or a combination of some or all of these products. The coagulation or curdling may be brought about by the enzyme action of rennet or pepsin, by lactic acid produced by bacterial action, or by a combination of both. After the initial draining, the cheese may be shaped in molds or presses, where additional moisture is removed. Cheese is classified on the basis of moisture content. Most cheese in this country is made from the milk of dairy cows, but the milk of other animals, chiefly goats and sheep, is also used.

Types of Cheese	Examples	Amount of Moisture
Fresh	Cottage, ricotta	80%
Soft	Brie, Camembert, cream	50–55%
Semisoft	Roquefort, blue, Gorgonzola, Limburger, Muenster	No more than 50%
Hard	Cheddar, Swiss, Edam, Colby, Gouda	39–41%
Very hard	Parmesan, Romano	Less than 32%

When milk is changed into cheese, the nutritional composition also changes. The milk is coagulated into curds (solids) and whey (liquid). When the whey is drained off, the water-soluble nutrients are largely drained off with it: milk sugar (lactose); the proteins lactalbumin and lactoglobulin; the minerals potassium, sodium, and magnesium; and the vitamins thiamin, riboflavin, niacin, vitamin B_6, pantothenic acid, biotin, and folacin. However, the solid curds then become a more concentrated source of the protein casein, and of fat, calcium, phosphorus, and vitamin A. The final cheese on the basis of weight may have eight to ten times as much of these as the original milk.

A second change in the composition of cheese takes place during ripening, or aging. Ripening is the holding of cheese

NUTRITIVE VALUE OF MILK (VARIOUS FORMS), YOGURT, CHEESE

	Amount	Energy Calories	Carbo-hydrate gm	Fat gm	Protein gm	Calcium mg	Phosphorus mg	Magnesium mg	Sodium mg
Breast milk	4 oz	92	11	5	2	40	17	5	18
Milk, homogenized	8 oz	150	12	8	8	291	228	33	120
low fat, 2%	8 oz	121	12	5	8	297	232	33	122
2% fat and protein	8 oz	135	14	8	10	352	276	+	+
1% fat and protein	8 oz	120	14	3	10	349	273	+	+
skim	8 oz	86	12	.4	8	302	247	28	126
Buttermilk, 2% fat	8 oz	99	12	2	8	285	219	27	257
Chocolate milk	8 oz	208	26	8.5	8	280	251	33	149
Chocolate dairy drink	8 oz	158	26	2.5	8	287	256	33	152
Evaporated milk	4 oz	169	13	10	9	329	255	30	133
Sweetened condensed	8 oz	982	166	27	24	868	775	78	389
Instant non-fat dry	3.2 oz	326	48	1	32	1120	896	107	499
With Vit. A & D reconstituted	8 oz	82	12	.2	8	280	224	27	125
Whole milk, dry	1 tbsp	40	3	2	2	73	62	7	30
Yogurt, plain, whole milk	8 oz	139	11	7	8	274	215	26	105
plain, skim milk	8 oz	127	17	.4	13	452	355	43	174
fruit	8 oz	231	43	2.5	10	345	271	33	133
Cheese, brick	1 oz	105	0	8	7	191	128	7	159
Brie	1 oz	95	0	8	6	52	53	+	178
Camembert	1 oz	85	0	7	6	110	98	6	239
Cheddar	1 oz	114	0	9	7	204	145	8	176
cottage, creamed	½ c	108	0	5	13	63	139	5	425
cottage, dry	½ c	62	0	.3	12	23	75	3	10
cream	1 oz	99	0	10	2	23	30	2	84
feta	1 oz	75	0	6	4	140	96	5	316
Cheese, Gouda	1 oz	101	0	8	7	198	155	8	+
Gruyere	1 oz	117	0	9	8	287	172	+	95
Monterey	1 oz	106	0	9	7	212	126	8	152
mozzarella	1 oz	80	0	6	5	147	105	5	106
Parmesan, grated	¼ c	129	0	8	12	390	229	14	528
provolone	1 oz	100	0	7	.7	214	141	8	248
ricotta, whole milk	½ c	214	0	16	16	254	194	14	104
Roquefort	1 oz	105	0	8	6	188	111	8	513
Swiss	1 oz	107	0	8	8	272	171	10	74
Process cheese, American	1 oz	106	0	9	6	174	211	6	406
Cheese food	1 oz	93	0	7	6	163	130	9	337
Cheese spread	1 oz	82	0	6	5	159	202	8	381

+ Probably present.
— No data.

Potassium mg	Iron mg	Zinc mg	Vitamin A IU	Vitamin E Tocopherol mg	Thiamin mg	Riboflavin mg	Niacin mg	Vitamin B-6 mg	Pantothenic Acid mg	Folacin mcg	Vitamin B-12 mcg	Cholesterol mg	Vitamin D IU
58	.1	.4	167	.7	.02	.05	.2	.01	.3	2	.05	+	+
370	.1	.9	307	.1	.1	.4	.2	.1	.8	12	.9	33	100
377	.1	1	500	—	.1	.4	.2	.1	.8	12	.9	18	100
+	.1	+	500	0	.1	.5	.2	+	+	+	+	18	100
+	.1	+	500	0	.1	.5	.2	+	+	+	+	10	100
406	.1	1	500	0	.1	.3	.2	.1	.8	13	.9	4	100
371	.1	1	81	0	.08	.4	.1	.08	.7	+	.5	9	—
417	.6	1	302	—	.09	.4	.3	.1	.7	12	.8	30	—
426	.6	1	500	—	.10	.4	.3	.1	.8	12	.9		—
382	.2	1	306	.2	.06	.4	.2	.06	.8	10	.2	37	—
1136	.6	2.9	1004	—	.03	1.3	.6	.16	2.3	34	+	104	—
1552	.3	4	2157	0	.38	1.6	.8	.31	2.9	45	3.6	17	400
388	.1	1	539	0	.09	.4	.2	.08	.7	11	.9	4	100
106	+	.3	74	+	.02	.1	+	.02	.1	3	.2	8	—
351	.1	1.3	279	.10	.06	.3	.2	.07	.9	17	.8	29	—
579	.2	2.2	16	0	.1	.5	.3	.12	1.5	28	1.4	4	—
442	.2	1.7	104	—	.08	.4	.2	.09	1.1	21	1.1	10	—
38	.1	.7	307	—	+	.1	.03	.02	.08	6	.4	27	0
43	.1	+	187	—	.02	.15	.11	.07	.19	18	.5	28	0
53	.1	.7	262	—	+	.14	.18	.06	.39	18	.4	20	0
28	.2	.9	300	.4	+	.11	.02	.02	.12	5	.2	30	0
88	.2	.4	171	.1	.02	.17	.13	.07	.22	13	.7	15	0
24	.2	.3	22	0	.02	.10	.11	.06	.12	10	.6	5	0
34	.3	.1	405	.3	+	.05	.03	.01	.08	4	.1	31	0
18	.2	.8	—	—	—	—	—	—	—	—	—	25	0
+	.1	1.1	183	+	+	.1	.02	.02	.1	6	+	32	0
23	+	+	346	+	.02	.08	.03	.02	.16	3	.45	31	0
23	.2	.8	269	—	—	.11	—	—	+	+	+	—	0
19	.1	.6	225	—	—	.07	.02	.01	.02	2	.19	22	0
30	.3	.9	199	—	—	.11	.09	.03	.15	2	+	22	0
39	.2	.9	231	—	—	.10	.04	.05	.14	3	.41	20	0
128	.5	1.4	602	+	.01	.24	.13	.03	+	+	.41	62	0
26	.1	.6	297	.3	—	.16	.21	.02	.49	14	.18	33	0
31	.1	1.1	240	—	—	.10	.03	.02	.12	2	.48	26	0
46	.1	.8	343	.3	—	.10	.02	—	.14	2	.20	27	0
79	.2	.7	259	—	—	.13	.04	—	.16	—	.32	18	0
69	.1	.7	223	—	.01	.12	.04	.06	.19	2	.11	16	0

under controlled conditions to allow chosen bacteria and enzymes to change the fresh curd into a cheese of specific flavor, texture, and appearance. Any remaining vitamin C is lost in the ripening, but some of the B-vitamins may be synthesized by the ripening organisms.

Nutritive Value of Cheese and Cheese Products

The nutritive values of natural cheese have the characteristics of the milk from which they were made, taking into account the losses in the whey. The preceding table gives the complete nutritive value of 1 ounce of the common cheeses as compared with an 8-ounce glass of milk.

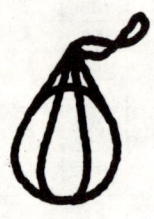

Cheese Standards

The aging or ripening of natural cheese continues even after they are ready for sale. The timing of the production and distribution of cheese must be carefully calculated to avoid excess ripening, spoilage, and waste. This is especially true of the soft cheeses and fresh cheese, such as cottage cheese. In modern food marketing, to counteract this natural course of events, techniques have been developed for processing and pasteurizing the ripened cheese to stop any further changes. Cheese is now manipulated into many products. These products have a long shelf and distribution life. The name on the package of such cheese and cheese products is the first clue as to their method of production, their composition, and their nutritive value. In order to be labeled by the name on the package the product has to meet a government standard. The following are the standards for some categories:

Cottage cheese is fresh cheese or curds, and it is an excellent protein food. Because acidified water is often used to wash the curds, some of the calcium of the milk is lost. The fat content must not be less than 4 percent milk fat.

Cottage cheese—low fat is fresh cheese as above and must contain from ½ to 2 percent milk fat.

Cottage cheese—dry curd is fresh cheese or curds as above and must contain less than ½ percent milk fat.

Pasteurized process cheese is made by combining and grinding several batches of natural cheese, adding an emulsifying agent, and then heating and mixing the cheese until smooth. The composition of process cheese is governed by a standard of identity which specifies what ingredients it must contain and that it be pasteurized. Its fat and moisture content must generally equal those of the cheese from which it is made.

Pasteurized process cheese food is made in a way similar to process cheese, but its composition is governed by a standard which permits the addition of skim milk, cream, and whey. It must not be more than 44 percent moisture and not less than 23 percent fat.

Pasteurized process cheese spread is also made in a way similar to process cheese and comes in many forms and flavors. Its composition is governed by a standard which permits the addition of skim milk, cream, whey, enzyme modified cheese, and emulsifiers. It must be between 44 and 60 percent moisture and not less than 20 percent fat.

Pasteurized process cheese product is made with skim milk cheese, cheese, and enzyme modified cheese solids. It is low in fat.

NOTE: The name on the package (process cheese, cheese food, cheese spread, cheese product) indicates a manufacturing change from natural cheese. Whereas the protein, calcium, and riboflavin values are major nutrient levels to watch when comparing these products to milk, the loss of some of the other nutrients, such as thiamin, may be just as important. People watching their weight and fat intake would be wise to note the fat content on the labels of these cheese products.

8.

Protein Foods: Meat, Poultry, Fish, Eggs, and Legumes

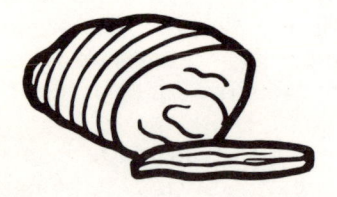

We are a nation of meat eaters, and our preference is more and more for the muscle meat of beef. Muscle meats are the roasts, steaks, chops, and ground meat from all the meat animals. Beef is a symbol of status and well-being to many of us. In 1976 125 pounds of beef were produced for each of us. This is a great credit to our agriculture and a bonus to our health—up to a point. And as beef consumption has gone up, pork, lamb, and veal consumption has gone down, which reflects a narrowing of our food likes. There has also been a general turning away from eating the heart, tongue, and organ meats of all the meat animals. Organ meats, because they are vital to the animal, are higher in minerals and vitamins than is muscle meat. Liver, including that from chicken, is an outstanding source of iron, vitamins, and trace minerals. Liver retains some popularity and most of its nutritional value as liverwurst, liver paté, and chopped liver.

NUTRIENTS IN MEAT

We usually think of meat as being a protein food, but like all other naturally occurring foods, it contributes a variety of nutrients. In the preceding chapter we saw that milk, although 87 percent water, is a main source of protein, calcium, phosphorus, and riboflavin. Meat from livestock and poultry, which is about 60 percent water, is a major source of protein, iron, zinc, vitamin B_{12}, vitamin B_6, riboflavin, niacin, and thiamin. Meat contains fat, but no carbohydrates; phosphorus, but little calcium. Only liver has lots of vitamin A.

Meat does not supply you with calcium, vitamin C, vitamin A, or vitamin D.

Protein of Meat

The proteins of meat have a high biological value, ranking in third place after egg and milk. (Biological values of proteins are given and explained in Chapter 3.) Meat proteins are complete proteins and can supplement the proteins of cereals and vegetables, which lack some essential amino acids. Even as small an amount as 1 ounce of meat added to a quite large serving of grain or vegetable will make up for this lack and increase the value of the grain and vegetable proteins. The age-old custom of eating meats and grains and vegetables in the same meal is an example of instinctive good nutrition.

Fats of Meat

Much has been written on the fat of meat, and much of what we know about the effect of diet on fat stores in the body comes from studying the feeding of animals for food. We have learned two main things. First, when pigs are fed peanuts or fats which are highly unsaturated, that is, softer and more oily, their fat is also more unsaturated. To a small extent the same is true of beef and lamb. Second, meat with a certain amount of marbling or visible fat in the muscle is more tender when cooked than meat with little marbling.

Most old cookbooks recommend that beef, game, or veal be larded before cooking. Larding involves inserting strips of fat into the muscle before cooking to improve the tenderness and flavor of roasted or pot-roasted meat. We don't have to do this to present-day beef because for the final days of feeding most animals are "finished," or "fattened" by being supplied with ample food and having their activity restricted. The animals put on weight, mostly as saturated fat. This is an advantage in cookery but not for our health. The amount of visible fat used to be one of the criteria for grading beef, but this has now been changed. (See page 125.)

Whereas the beef animal is fattened for tenderness, the pork animal has been selectively bred to reduce the fat in the meat and is fed to produce leaner meat. So in today's meat supply there is little difference in the protein and fat content of muscle meats from all meat animals. You will get as much protein from poultry, but less fat, if you do not eat the skin.

The fats of meats are both saturated and unsaturated. Since cholesterol is one of the substances of the nervous system it is also present in meat. Meat contains just a small amount of linoleic acid, an essential fatty acid. The fats of meat we eat are in their biological form; that is, they still contain the vitamins and trace minerals essential for their formation in the living animal. Much of our food fat and oil (such as salad oil) is stripped of all trace minerals and vitamins and is as refined a source of calories as sugar. Whether or not this makes any difference in their use by the body we don't know.

In the table that follows, you can compare the protein, fat, cholesterol value of the major protein foods.

Phosphorus-Calcium Imbalance

Meats contain phosphorus but very little calcium. For this reason, if you are following one of the many high-protein diets written about in the popular press and you are eating a large amount of meat for its protein and not getting an adequate supply of calcium from milk, cheese, hard water, or canned fish bones, you risk losing some of the calcium in your bones.

Meat is also a good source of magnesium, another major mineral.

Iron

Meat has a higher iron content than milk and most other foods. Iron is the mineral needed to make oxygen-carrying hemoglobin in your blood. You don't need a very large amount daily because your body recycles as much as it can, but you lose some every day. Many foods show a high iron content when they are analysed chemically, but in many cases all this iron is not available to you. Either it is not extracted from the food during digestion, or else it comes in a form your body

CALORIES, PROTEIN, FAT, CHOLESTEROL AND CARBOHYDRATE CONTENT OF MAJOR PROTEIN FOODS

	Amount	Calories	Protein gm	Total Fat gm	Poly-unsaturated Fat gm	Saturated Fat gm	Cholesterol mgm	Carbo-hydrate gm
Milk, whole	8-oz glass	150	8	8	.3	5	33	12
Milk, skim	8-oz glass	86	8	.4	.1	.3	4	12
Cheddar cheese	1 ounce	114	7	9	.3	6	30	—
Beef, lean & marble	3½ ounces	266	30	15	.3	7	91	0
Pork	3½ ounces	240	28	13	.8	5	88	0
Lamb	3½ ounces	260	27	16	.2	10	100	0
Veal	3½ ounces	213	33	8	.4	4	99	0
Chicken ½ light ½ dark No Skin	3½ ounces	182	30	6	1	2	85	0
Turkey ½ light ½ dark	3½ ounces	188	32	6	1	2	89	0
Salmon	3½ ounces	180	27	7	.1	1	35	0
* Tuna, canned	3 ounces	170	24	7	.7	2	50	0
Fish, white	3½ ounces	170	25	7	—	—	60	0
Shrimp	3 ounces	100	20	1	+	—	150	0
Lobster	⅔ cup	95	19	2	+	—	85	0
Eggs, large	2	160	12	12	1.4	3.4	504	0
Legumes, cooked	¾ cup	165	9	1.5			0	27
Peanuts	¼ cup	210	9	18	5	4	0	7
Peanut butter	2 tbsp	190	9	17	5	4	0	6
Corn oil (reference fat)	1 tbsp	120	0	14	8	1.7	0	0

All meats and fish are cooked and trimmed of visible fat.
* Tuna, 3½-oz can, drained.

cannot take through the intestinal walls. The iron in meat is completely available. It is commonly thought that the natural red color of some meats is related to blood and that these meats are superior sources of protein and iron for blood building than the lighter meats. This is not so. The red color of some meats comes from myoglobin, which is just one of the proteins of red meat. The pink meats veal and pork and the white and dark meats of poultry are just as good sources of protein and almost as high in iron as red meat.

B-Vitamins

You can get many of the B-vitamins from vegetables, legumes, and cereals, but these foods cannot provide vitamin B_{12}, because it does not exist in the plant kingdom. Since animals and human beings need it, we must get it from animal foods—meat, eggs, fish, and milk. Until 1948 the only known treatment for pernicious anemia was the elusive factor present in liver or liver extract, which we now know is vitamin B_{12}. Meat, especially liver, is also one of the best sources of vitamin B_6. This vitamin is also present in a few vegetables and cereals, but since it can be destroyed by high-heat processing, fresh meat and fish are our best sources. The need for and the role these vitamins B_6 and B_{12} play in our health has been unraveled in just the last few years. Having a serving of liver at least once a week is one of the best ways of getting these vitamins, along with a natural supply of iron and zinc.

Riboflavin and niacin are two other B-vitamins you can count on getting from a serving of meat; and tryptophan, one of the essential amino acids, also present in good supply in meat, can be converted by your body to supplement the supply of niacin if there is too little niacin in your diet to meet your needs. Organ meats contain more thiamin than muscle meats do, with the exception of pork, which is the best meat source of thiamin. Some thiamin is lost in cooking and in processing.

Trace Minerals

Iron is the most important trace mineral you get from meat. Meat also provides copper, which works along with iron in blood making and in releasing energy from glucose. Other trace minerals found in meats are zinc, manganese, selenium, chromium, and molybdenum. Their function in the miraculous and complicated business of making cells and releasing energy for living is covered in Chapter 4.

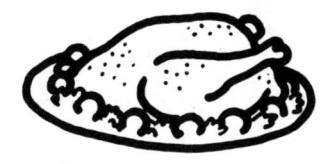

POULTRY AND FISH

Poultry gives you as much nutrition as the other meats. The main difference between the two is the amount of fat in proportion to the protein. A serving of poultry without skin is as high in protein, but somewhat lower in fat and, therefore, in calories. An overall reduction in the amount of fat we eat seems to have a beneficial effect on our health. The composition of the fat also seems to make a difference. The fat of poultry is slightly less saturated, which is more desirable. (See the table on page 119.) You can compare the other small differences in mineral and vitamin content of the two groups in the table of nutritive values of protein foods (page 122).

The old concept of fish as a brain food is not valid, but most of the facts about meat apply to fish. The protein of fish is as good for you as the protein of meat. Fish have less fat than meats. Some shellfish have no fat as such; it is present in the form of cholesterol and sterols.

Fish is a good source of phosphorus, and the bones of canned salmon and sardines are a source of calcium. Fish also contain iron and copper and other trace minerals. Ocean fish have two additional trace minerals, iodine and fluorine. The contribution fish makes to your daily vitamin B needs are about the same as meat. Raw fish, however, has an enzyme that puts thiamin out of action, so fish should be cooked if you are counting on it to supply thiamin. Vitamin A concentrated in the liver of fish is used in the manufacture of vitamin supplements, not as a food.

NUTRITIVE VALUE OF HIGH PROTEIN FOODS AS EATEN COOKED

	Amount	Energy Calories	Carbo-hydrate (gm)	Fat (gm)	Protein (gm)	Calcium (mg)	Phosphorus (mg)	Magnesium (mg)	Sodium (mg)
Milk, whole	8 oz	150	12	8	8	291	228	33	120
Beef	3½ oz	266	0	15	30	10	191	21	60
Beef liver	3½ oz	238	6	11	28	11	472	14	183
Lamb	3½ oz	260	0	16	27	8	211	23	67
Pork	3½ oz	240	0	13	28	8	228	23	68
Veal	3½ oz	213	0	8	33	10	260	22	65
Chicken	3½ oz	182	0	6	30	13	253	19	75
Turkey	3½ oz	188	0	6	32	8	251	19	90
Fish, white	3½ oz	170	0	5	29	31	273	24	108
Lobster	⅔ c	95	—	2	19	65	191	22	200
Salmon	3½ oz	180	0	7	27	259*	409	30	115
Shrimps	3 oz	100	1	1	21	98	224	48	—
Tuna, canned in oil	3 oz	170	0	7	24	7	199	24	—
Eggs	2	160	1	12	12	56	180	12	292
Black-eyed peas (frozen)	¾ c	169	31	—	12	32	218	—	50
Garbanzo (chick pea)	¾ c	165	27	2	9	67	149	49	+
Kidney (Pinto) beans	¾ c	173	32	1	11	56	209	—	3
Lentils	¾ c	158	29	—	12	38	178	—	—
Lima beans (fresh/frozen)	¾ c	126	24	—	8	26	114	61	129
dried, cooked	¾ c	197	37	1	12	41	220	55	28
Pea beans, dried, cooked	¾ c	169	30	1	11	71	210	56	10
canned, vegetarian	¾ c	230	45	1	12	130	231	50	647
canned with pork	¾ c	233	36	5	12	103	176	70	886
Peas, fresh or frozen	¾ c	83	14	—	6	23	103	28	154
dried, split	¾ c	173	31	—	12	17	133	—	20
Soybeans, dried, cooked	¾ c	176	15	8	15	98	242	360	3
Soybean curd	4 oz	86	3	4	9	154	151	—	8
Soybean-textured patties	2½ oz	182	7	11	14	20	—	0	822
Peanut butter	2 tbsp	190	4	17	9	10	120	50	150

* Canned.
+ Probably present.
— No data.
Meats have visible fat removed.
Chicken—no skin, half dark, half white meat.

mg	mg	mg	IU	mg	mg	mg	mg	mg	mg	mcg	mcg	mg	IU
Potassium	Iron	Zinc	Vitamin A	Vitamin E	Thiamin	Riboflavin	Niacin	Vitamin B-6	Pantothenic Acid	Folacin	Vitamin B-12	Vitamin C	Vitamin D
370	.1	.9	307	.1	.1	.4	.2	.1	.8	12	.9	2	100
261	4	6	50	1	.1	.4	4.5	.4	.5	4	2	0	0
376	9	10	56070	3	.3	4.3	17	.8	8.1	308	84	28	14
317	2	5	—	.2	.2	.3	7.6	.3	.6	4	2.8	0	0
326	4	4	—	.2	1	.3	4.4	.5	.5	5	1.2	0	0
246	3.3	4	—	+	.2	.3	7.2	.5	.9	3	2.5	0	0
377	1.5	2	132	.4	.1	.1	8.8	.5	1	3	.4	0	0
367	1.8	3	—	—	.1	.2	7.6	—	—	—	—	0	0
403	1	1	180	1.2	.1	.1	3	.4	.3	—	1	2	0
180	.8	2.2	—	1.7	.1	.1	—	—	—	—	—	0	0
441	1	.9	160	1.4	.2	.1	9.8	.7	1.3	—	4	0	314
104	2.6	2	50	.4	—	—	1.5	—	.2	2	—	0	0
301	1.6	1	70	.5	—	.1	10	.4	.3	2	2.2	0	300
130	2	1.4	520	1	.1	.3	—	.1	1.7	49	1.2	0	54
438	3.7	1.7	220	—	.5	.1	1.8	—	—	—	0	1.2	0
+	3.1	1.8	23	—	.15	—	.9	.2	.6	57	0	0	0
505	3.4	1.7	8	—	.1	—	1.1	—	—	—	0	0	0
374	3.1	1.5	30	—	.1	.1	1	—	—	—	0	0	0
543	2.1	1.2	293	—	.1	—	1.3	.2	.3	44	0	22	0
872	4.4	1.2	—	—	.2	.1	1	.3	.3	—	0	0	0
592	3.8	1.4	—	.3	.2	.1	1	.2	.3	12	0	0	0
512	3.8	2	113	.3	.1	.1	1.1	.2	.3	45	0	2	0
402	3.4	2.5	247	0	.2	.1	1.1	—	.2	—	—	4	0
162	2.3	.9	720	30	.32	.10	2	.15	.39	30	0	16	0
444	2.6	1.7	60	—	.23	.14	1.4	.04	.44	—	0	0	0
729	3.7	—	37	—	.29	.12	.8	.36	.76	100	0	0	0
50	2.3	—	0	—	.07	.04	.1	—	—	—	—	0	0
—	3	0	0	0	.23	.26	7	.20	0	0	2.4	—	0
220	.6	.9	0	6	.02	.02	4.2	.1	.4	26	0	0	0

HOW MUCH MEAT SHOULD YOU EAT?

You can see from the table that you do not get calcium from meat and that when you drink milk for calcium, you also get a good supply of protein. If you consume enough milk or cheese, all you need is one serving of meat or an alternate protein food; grain foods and vegetables also supply protein.

But first, what is a serving? Nutritionists usually consider 3 to 3½ ounces of cooked meat with all the visible fat cut off to be one serving of meat. This equals 4 to 5 ounces of raw lean meat. Menus in some restaurants advertise 8- to 12-ounce steaks or cuts of prime ribs of beef. This may be all right as an occasional treat, but remember that you are eating two servings of calories and fat, and more protein than you need.

How much of the protein in extra large servings of meat is used as protein? In the chapter on protein and amino acids, the synthesis of a protein is outlined as simply as possible; it is a very complex process, however. One thing we know about the process is that it goes on at quite a rapid rate following a meal, and then it slows. If not enough protein is eaten and not enough amino acids are therefore available for synthesis, the process will stop. On the other hand, if a lot of protein is eaten, the process stops as soon as the body's immediate needs are met. The extra amino acids are not stored as amino acids for future use. They are changed into fat and packed away just for their energy. The part that made them valuable as amino acids is discarded.

It is much wiser on a day-to-day and meal-to-meal basis to make more economical use of the protein foods by including them in each meal. Two small hamburgers, one at lunch and one at dinner, will be much better used for protein replacement than one double-sized one consumed at one eating. The practice of adding soy bean protein to hamburgers to make them bigger is an example of a wasteful use of this protein, and encourages overconsumption of food as well.

In the early part of this century, less meat per capita was produced and available to the population than is the case today. As we near the end of this century, our population may face a return to consumption of less meat per person. It is to be hoped that meat will still be available to those in lower income brackets. There may come a time in the future when high-protein foods will have to be used more economically in combination with grains and vegetables, especially legumes. Our understanding of the chemistry of nutrition will help us balance all the nutrients involved. And the consequent lowering of fat in our diets will help in weight control and health maintenance.

CONSUMER PROTECTION

Inspection Stamp for Wholesomeness

Before any meat can be sold as food, it must bear the USDA's little round stamp of approval. We never see it on meat in the supermarket because it is stamped on the outer fat layer of the carcass in meat-packing plants. This fat is trimmed off by the butcher when the meat is packaged into retail cuts. You will find the seal on every canned and packaged product that contains meat. The seal was established by the Federal Meat Inspection Act in 1906. It means that the animal or bird was in good health and was slaughtered and processed under inspected sanitary conditions. The scope of this legislation was broadened in 1967 with the passage of the Wholesome Meat Act.

Grading

There have been some recent changes in beef grading. When these changes were first proposed, some consumers feared that an attempt at fraud was in the making. This was not the case, but the reaction did show how little most of us know about how our meat supply is protected. Meat grading was established in 1927. The qualifications for certain grades have been updated every seven to ten years, as breeding and feeding have developed animals with more tender meat. The three top grades of beef, veal, and lamb are Prime, Choice, and Good; for pork the grades are U.S. 1, U.S. 2, and U.S. 3. There are grades below these, but the lower-grade meats are usually used in processed meat and "convenience" products. The meat in the lower grades is just as wholesome but tougher and less satisfactory for home cooking.

One of the features of prime meat is the amount of fat that runs through the meat as light streaks or "marble." While this fat assures us of tender meat, too much fat does not seem to be good for us. Because present-day meat is bred and raised to be much more tender than it was years ago, and especially because of the question of fat in relation to health, the grading standards of beef were changed in 1976. Beef with less marbling that would have been graded by the old standard "Choice" can now be graded "Prime."

The best of beef formerly graded as "Good" will be a lower-fat beef grade as "Choice," and that at the lower end of the "Good" will be graded "Standard." The remaining, though smaller amount, still graded as "Good" will be a lower fat and less expensive grade for sale as fresh meat.

In 1965, a new grading of beef based on yield of meat in relationship to fat was begun. With the 1976 regulation, all beef will be graded for both quality (palatability) and yield (percentage of edible meat). Other qualifications that beef must meet to be given a top grade are color, texture, firmness of the lean meat, and age of the animal.

Grading of meat is not required by law. Meat packers pay for the government agents, who are already on the job to inspect the meat, to grade it. If the grade is advertised, however, the meat must be of that grade.

Uniform Retail Meat Identity Standard

Another change the meat industry made recently was the adoption of the Uniform Retail Meat Identity Standard. This is an agreement to call the same cut of meat the same name whether it is sold in Maine or California. Each cut of meat is to be labeled in a uniform way. From the more than 1000 names that were being used across the country, 300 standard names have been chosen. The label will tell the kind of meat, such as beef, pork, veal and lamb; the name of the part of the animal from which it was cut, such as rib, loin, leg, and shoulder; and finally the retail cut, such as steak, roast, and chop.

With the help of standard names you can always be sure of what you are buying. Since some cuts are higher in fat than others, you will also get indirect nutritional information if you wish to purchase the lower fat cuts.

Ground beef is one of the most popular and most used of all forms of meat. In 1976 almost 40 percent of all the beef eaten was ground. Under the new code, meat labeled as ground beef must be pure beef from only muscle meat. The label may also add whether it is from the chuck, round, or sirloin. Retailers adopting the new standard will list the percentage of fat in the product or the ratio of fat to meat. Ground beef can vary in leanness from 90 percent meat with 10 percent fat to 70 percent meat with 30 percent fat. There is a law that prohibits more than 30 percent fat in ground beef.

Perishability

Meat is a very perishable food. For this reason, procuring fresh meat, poultry, and fish and keeping it from spoilage have always been a challenge to the consumer. In some parts of the world, even today, the local butcher obtains supplies for his market stall or store directly from the farmer every day or every week, and each morning the person who does the cooking for the household buys meat there for that day. In other places the challenge is met by meat processors and refrigerated and frozen meat products for supermarkets and homes.

We have two legacies from the older methods for keeping a supply of meat on hand without spoilage. One is cured meats, such as corned beef, dried beef, ham, and bacon. The other is 200 or more varieties of sausage. Sausage making used to be an art of butchers, who had their own recipes for the meats and spices to be used in such products as pork sausage, veal sausage, beef-and-pork sausage, and many others. It was an art that developed out of economy, since to make sausages he could use the tougher meat and trimmings from prime cuts of the whole animal. Because most sausages are now made by meat companies and not by local butchers who are known and trusted, consumers question the ingredients used. In 1967 a bill was passed that required that the ingredients in a food product be listed on the label: "The ingredients shall be listed by common or usual name in order of decreasing predominance by weight." You can now read the contents on the label.

Many by-products that were formerly used in sausages are needed by the medical profession. Many organs and blood are used in pharmaceutical products. For example, the glandular meats are sources of hormones. Each of the 5 million diabetics in the country requires the insulin from about 26 head of cattle to keep well for one year. Even the supply of liver, which is such a good food, is divided between food and medical uses. So it is very unlikely that organ meats that are being used for these valuable new products would end up in sausages.

Sausage Labels

Under the present laws of meat inspection, both the formula for the sausage and the wording on the label must be approved by the government before the sausage can be made. The animals used for meat are inspected and the meat must be handled under approved conditions. Fresh or uncured sausages are highly perishable, so you usually find them in the frozen food cabinets in the supermarket. They are raw fresh meat, and if not frozen must be used within a day. If they are frozen, keep them frozen until used. Some of the frozen ones have been "browned" by the meat packer and must be heated enough before serving to complete the cooking. They are treated with vitamin C to prevent changes in the flavor of the fat. The thiamin content can be diminished by long or poor storage.

Many sausages are cured so they will keep. The most popular, of course, is the frankfurter, hot dog, or wiener, whichever name you prefer. Some sausages are smoked, some are fully cooked, some are both cooked and smoked, and some are dried. The exact ingredient content and processing vary from brand to brand. But there are standards or accepted recipes established by the USDA that state what and how much of the basic ingredients may be used. The label will tell you.

Sausages labeled simply as frankfurters, bologna, knockwurst, cooked salami, and other cooked sausages can contain only muscle meat, no more than 30 percent fat, 10 percent added water, and 2 percent corn syrup. The muscle meat may be beef, pork, veal, lamb, and up to 15 percent chicken. Because they have added spices, the FDA has ruled that frankfurters and other cooked sausages can no longer be labeled "all meat," "pure meat," or "100 percent meat." So frankfurters, for example, are labeled "meat" and are usually made of beef, pork, and seasonings; sometimes they are labeled "beef" and are only beef with seasonings.

Frankfurters, bologna, and similar cooked sausages with by-products or variety meats are so labeled. These must contain 15 percent muscle meat, no more than 30 percent fat, 10 percent added water, and 2 percent corn syrup. The name of any additional meats must be given. These are usually heart and tongue, which are actually muscle meats. Frankfurters, bologna, and similar cooked sausages with by-products, which also contain non-meat binders, must contain no more than 30 percent fat; 10 percent added water; 2 percent corn syrup as in the above products but can contain 2 percent soy protein or 3½ percent nonmeat binders such as nonfat dry milk. These must be distinctly on the label as well as in the name; for example, "frankfurters with byproducts and nonfat dry milk added."

Liver products including sausage, paté, spread, and loaf, must contain 30 percent liver. Liverwurst must contain pork and 30 percent liver. There are many more meat products that must meet the requirement of established USDA standards before they can be sold.

Use of Nitrates and Nitrites

Sodium nitrite may be among the ingredients you will find listed on the package of ham, corned beef, bacon, sausages, and other cured meats. This salt, known as Chile saltpeter, and its cousin, sodium nitrate, along with sodium chloride (table salt), have been used throughout the centuries to keep meat from spoiling. The word *sausage* is derived from the Latin word *salsus*, meaning "salted." Before we had modern refrigeration and freezing, salting was the major way of keeping meat. The most deadly of all food poisoning, botulism toxin, develops in spoiled meat. Even a trace of this toxin in food can cause paralysis and death. The sodium nitrite in the salt mixture used in curing meat prevents the development of this deadly toxin. This is really why you may find sodium nitrite in the list of ingredients on cured meats, but it does other things as well. It prevents fat from becoming rancid or developing an off-taste, produces the popular cured flavor, and produces a pretty pink color. There are those who misconstrue these reactions and say the sodium nitrite is used mainly to keep the red color, but the fact that it produces an attractive color is incidental to its action as a preservative.

In the last few years there has been a great concentration of research on factors in food and the environment which might cause cancer. Among the substances found to produce cancer in rats were compounds of nitrates and protein. This occurred at very high levels of intake, but it nevertheless cast a suspicion on the safety of cured meats. The result has been a change in the way meat is cured, and sodium nitrate is no longer used in most cured meats. It is used in certain fermented sausages and dry-cured products. In fermented sausages, the lactic acid produced by fermentation aids in preserving the product. In other cured meats, as an added precaution, the amount of nitrite used has been reduced to the minimum needed to do the job.

Research also showed that harmful compounds were more easily formed at a high temperature, such as that used in frying bacon. So the amount of sodium nitrite used for curing bacon has been further reduced, and vitamin C is added to block the harmful reaction. Cured meats are still on the market, and their safety is constantly monitored.

Ham Labels

The U.S. Department of Agriculture and the FDA regulate the curing agents that can be used in the production of corned beef and ham. Ham must also meet another standard. It must not weigh more after the processing than the fresh meat weighed. Ham with any increase up to 10 percent must be labeled as having water added. If there is more than a 10 percent increase it has to be labeled as imitation ham. In addition to the list of ingredients used in curing, ham labels provide information on how to keep it to avoid any risk of spoilage. Most of today's hams must be refrigerated. Labels of such ham say "fully cooked" and "keep refrigerated." Further cooking improves the flavor but is not necessary. Other hams are not cooked and are labeled "cook-before-eating." They must be refrigerated and cooked to an internal temperature of 160° F before eating.

Canned hams weighing more than 1½ pounds have been fully cooked in a hot water bath to pasteurize them. This process plus the curing preserves the ham only if the ham is stored under refrigeration. Canned hams weighing less than 1½ pounds are pressure-cooked and can be stored on the shelf like other canned foods. Prosciutto ham is not fully cooked but is cooked sufficiently so that it is safe to eat.

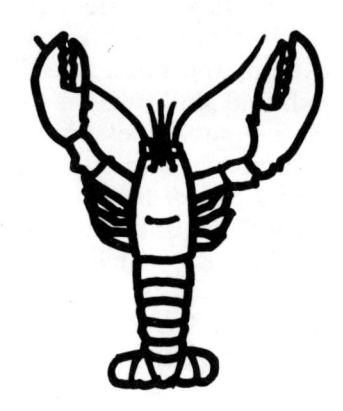

Inspection and Labeling of Poultry and Fish

In 1959 the Poultry Products Inspection Act was passed. It ruled that all chickens, turkeys, ducks, and Cornish game hens produced in one state and sold in another must be certified by federal inspectors for wholesomeness and production under sanitary conditions. Poultry grading (like meat grading) is done at the time of inspection. Although grading is requested and paid for by the producer, 99 percent of the poultry sold is government graded. The grades are A, B, and C. They are based on such criteria as appearance, skin tears, crooked breast bones, and amount of meat on the frame. Only grade A birds are sold fresh or fresh-frozen. The B and C grades are used in products where shape and appearance do not matter. The wholesomeness seal is like that for other meat. The grade is on a shield on the label.

If poultry is frozen, or frozen and thawed, it must be so labeled. If any ingredients have been added they must be indicated on the wrapping. This applies mostly to turkeys that have had a basting liquid of broth, butter, or oil injected into the meat. The type of oil, if used, must be stated. Canned chicken and turkey must meet government standards for the amount of meat in the can and contain only allowed ingredients, which have to be listed on the label. Packaged products in clear plastic wrapping come under similar regulations.

Whereas the Department of Agriculture inspects and grades meat and poultry, the Department of Commerce provides inspection and grading services for the fish and shellfish industry. Products that meet official standards can show the grade on the label along with a statement that packing was done under government inspection. In addition, shrimps, clams, oysters and other shellfish are graded as to size. Much of the fish and shellfish we eat is canned or packaged and frozen, or in "convenience" products. These products have to meet rigid "standards of identity" set by the FDA. For example, what goes into a can of tuna is spelled out in the regulations, as are the variety of tuna, the form (solid, chunk, flake), the amount of salt, what oil or liquid may be added, and even the time and temperature of the processing. There are similar standards for frozen and frozen breaded products. For example, a product labeled "lightly breaded shrimp" must be 65 percent shrimp by weight.

As these products must meet the standard before they are allowed to be put on the store shelves, it has not seemed necessary to put the information on the label. But now many companies are listing ingredients and giving nutrition information on the labels to inform consumers that the products were subject to such regulations.

Imported fish products must meet the same standards as domestic products before they are approved for sale.

Labeling Poultry and Processed Meat

In 1967 the Wholesome Meat Act was passed. By this act the government not only required that all meat be inspected for wholesomeness, as had been the law since 1906, but that the labels on federally inspected meat and poultry products be truthful, accurate, and informative. The label as well as the product must pass inspection.

What the Label Must Have

Simple or common name, or a descriptive name that tells what ingredients other than meat are present.
USDA inspection stamp or shield.
List of ingredients in descending order by weight.
Information on how to care for the products, such as whether refrigeration is needed.
A statement that the product is "fully cooked" (otherwise it should be cooked).
Windows in bacon packages that show 70 percent of a full slice.
Weight of the product without the package.
Name and address of the manufacturer.
Nutrition information if any nutrition claim is made in advertising or promotion.

What the Label May Have

Nutrition information, even though no claims are made in advertising.

Freshness dating in one of three ways: date the product was packaged; "pull" date on which the product must be removed from sale; expiration date, or date after which the product should not be eaten.

The manufacturer or producer has done a great deal to ensure you a safe and nutritious product. But you must read the label so that you will know how to store and cook the product.

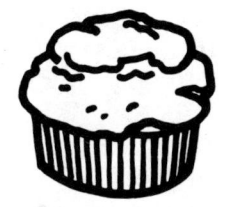

EGGS

While beef is the protein food that has the highest status in our society, the egg is perhaps the most downgraded. Yet the egg is one of the best of our protective and naturally occurring foods. Eggs are an excellent source of protein, iron, sulphur, and vitamin A. They are a good source of all the B-vitamins and phosphorus, along with some vitamin D and calcium. Eggs, like milk, are a food designed by nature to support life, so we can assume they contain all the trace minerals that we are learning about today. The only nutrient they lack is vitamin C.

Protein and Fat Content

Eggs are about half protein and half fat. In one large egg there are 6.5 grams of protein and 6 grams of fat. When you break an egg, it looks about half white and half yolk, so some people imagine that the white is the protein half and the yolk the fat half. This is not so. Egg white contains about half the protein (3 grams), and no fat. The white is high in riboflavin but contains no thiamin, and the minerals are in the yolk. Raw egg white also contains a substance called avidin that inactivates biotin, one of the B-vitamins, so egg white should be cooked before being eaten. The small amount eaten raw in some desserts is of no concern, however.

Egg yolk is extremely nutritious. It contains the other three grams or so of protein. The total proteins of egg white and yolk rank second only to human milk in supplying the amino acids in a ratio closest to the pattern of our needs.

The Cholesterol Controversy

The value of eggs as a food has been the subject of much publicity and much misinformation, centered on their fat and cholesterol content. An egg yolk contains about the same amount of fat as a half tablespoon (or pat) of margarine (6 grams). The fat of egg contains both saturated (1.7 grams) and polyunsaturated (.7 grams) fats. One of the unsaturated fats is linoleic acid, the only fatty acid essential to our health. Egg yolk contains other fatlike substances, among which are lecithin and cholesterol. Egg yolk is high in cholesterol—one egg yolk contains 252 milligrams.

When a person eats a meal that is high in cholesterol the level of cholesterol in the blood goes up. In a normal person, it goes down again from 4 to 6 hours later. From 5 to 7 percent of our population does not have this back-to-normal drop in cholesterol. Studies show that these people are likely to have fat deposits forming in their arteries, and this predisposes to heart disease. By measuring the level of cholesterol in the blood, doctors have a way of predicting if a person is likely to develop heart disease of this type. Cholesterol itself does not cause heart disease. Unless you have been tested several times and have been found to have a high level of cholesterol in your blood even though you have had nothing to eat or drink for 12 hours there is no reason to feel that eating eggs in normal amounts will cause narrowing of your heart arteries.

Other Nutrients

Iron

Eggs, like meat, are an excellent source of iron in usable form. They are especially valuable for babies. Babies, after three months, have usually used up the iron stores they are born with. Egg yolk is a made-to-order source of iron for them. It is also an excellent source at the other end of the age span. For older people, who may have trouble chewing meat, eggs are also an excellent source of protein and other nutrients.

Calcium

Unfortunately most of the egg's calcium is in the shell; the remaining small amount in the yolk is well absorbed and utilized. In some cultures, washed and dried shells are pounded to a powder and added to pasta and breads to improve the calcium content of these foods.

Phosphorus

Eggs are high in phosphorus and, like meat, if eaten without some calcium in your diet can produce an imbalance of these two elements. In many traditional recipes, eggs and milk (for calcium) are frequent companions, illustrating the nutritional wisdom of recipes handed down through time.

All Vitamins Except C

Eggs are an excellent source of vitamin A in a readily usable form. Eggs rank next to liver among the few foods that supply us with vitamin A already formed. Food surveys show that teenagers in America, especially girls, have low intakes of iron and vitamin A, both easily obtained by eating eggs. Eggs can be counted on to contribute a fair share of each of the B-vitamins, thiamin, riboflavin, niacin, pantothenic acid, folacin, B_6 and B_{12}. But they are not a source of vitamin C (ascorbic acid).

Consumer Protection

Inspection under state and federal regulations falls under the Egg Products Inspection Act, which guarantees that eggs in the shell and all commercial egg products are clean, wholesome, and safe to eat. Eggs are graded on their interior quality and the condition of their shells. Shells must be clean and not cracked. The interior quality is judged by holding the egg to a light. For the egg to be Grade AA or A (the quality found for sale in the shell), the yolk should be round and the white firm. Grade B eggs go into commercial products and may be sold as canned, frozen, or dried whites or yolks. There is some evidence that the chemical nature of the cholesterol of eggs is changed by the drying process.

All commercial egg products must meet FDA regulations as to wholesomeness. Commercial egg products are used in bakeries, the manufacture of mayonnaise, and other products. About 13 percent of all eggs produced go into "convenience" foods. The eggs you buy in the store are graded according to size as well as quality. The sizes are based on the weight of a dozen eggs, and are jumbo (30 ounces), extra large (27 ounces), large (24 ounces), medium (21 ounces), and small (18 ounces). Egg cartons do not have nutritional information on them. Brown and white eggs have the same nutritional value; they are just laid by different breeds of hen. Similarly, dark yellow egg yolks are no better nutritionally than light yellow ones. Eggs are a perishable protein food and should be refrigerated. Egg cartons may have open dating.

HIGH-PROTEIN PLANT FOODS

You don't have to get protein from animal foods. In fact, most of the world's population get most of their protein from plant foods. The best plant food sources are cereals and legumes. These are the seeds of plants, and they contain the nutrients needed for new plants to grow. Other vegetables supply some protein, while fruits contain practically none.

Processed vegetable products must meet government standards (see page 151). Many canned and frozen legumes, including such widely used "convenience" products as pork and beans and chili con carne, carry nutritional information on their labels. If soy protein concentrate is added to ground meat, the product must be so labeled.

Legumes

Legumes (sometimes referred to as *pulses* when dried) include all the various peas and beans one finds around the world. Often the same vegetables have different names in different places. Legumes are a major source of protein after animal food. Perhaps they should be considered as a food group apart from meat for three reasons.

- Many people today are interested in vegetarian diets.
- One concern of people interested in vegetarianism is the need to provide protein for our worldwide populations, now as well as in the future. Since legumes are less expensive to produce, in terms of energy and land use, they are a less wasteful source of protein.

✔ Considering legumes as replacements for all animal foods is not nutritionally sound for all nutrients. Legumes are a low-fat source of protein, which is very desirable, but their protein, with the exception of soybean and garbanzo protein, is of lower biological value.

Protein Content

The legumes vary in their protein content and in the value of that protein. When a mature pea or bean has been dried and then cooked, it is a much more concentrated source than the fresh pea or bean. This can be seen in the table on page 156. But even when fresh, most legumes have protein of a useful although not high biological value. In Chapter 3 we pointed out that the biological value of a food depends on the amount and number of the eight essential amino acids present in that food. With the exception of garbanzos (also called chick peas or Bengal grams) and soybeans, which contain all the essential amino acids, the legumes lack at least one amino acid, usually methionine.

In recent years much has been learned about the process of protein synthesis in our bodies. One of the most important things is that protein synthesis will take place as long as all the amino acids are present at the same time. In the digestive process, all the protein foods of a meal are mixed together, and the mixture of amino acids from them is absorbed together. We can, therefore, use complementary or supplementary foods.

By analyzing foods for their amino acid content, it was found that red beans are low in methionine but have a good supply of lysine and tryptophan. Corn, on the other hand, has an amino acid content the other way around. When eaten together the total amount of amino acids is about the same as you would get from meat. The amino acids of the corn and beans—a common combination in Mexican and other types of cooking—provide a combined mixture for maximum protein synthesis from the foods. And the carbohydrate provides a source of calories that prevents the amino acids from being used as a source of energy.

The balance of amino acids needed for making protein is very exacting, and an excess of some can increase the need for others. For that reason, you should not make your own amino acid mixtures or supplement your foods with the synthetic products that are now sold in health food stores. The simplest way to supplement the protein of the legumes is the one with the greatest taste appeal and acceptance, and that is by the addition of milk, cheese, meat, fish, poultry, or eggs and the whole grains. Recipe books are filled with such nutritionally sound and good combinations.

Cooking Requirements

Legumes are more like cereals than meat, since they are carbohydrate foods and, except for soybeans and peanuts, contain little fat. The carbohydrate is in a complex form and difficult to digest. For this reason, legumes should be well cooked. The dried forms especially require long, slow cooking to break down the carbohydrate so that the vegetable will be digested and all its nutrients made available. Unfortunately, the long cooking also results in a fairly substantial loss of the thiamin, which is destroyed by heat. Riboflavin and niacin are less affected.

Some legumes (lima beans, pea beans, kidney beans, soy beans, and fava beans) contain toxic substances. One of these inhibits the action of trypsin, one of the enzymes that digest protein, and therefore interferes with protein digestion. Another affects the blood. Cooking puts both toxins out of action.

Legumes, like cereals, are fairly high in phosphorus, some of which is bound in a compound called phytic acid or phytate. This compound affects the usability of some of the minerals. Phytic acid combines with both calcium and iron. When looking at a table of food values like that on page 156, the legumes seem to be a good source of iron. However some of this iron may be bound with phytates which you do not digest, so some iron may not be available for your use. In a similar manner phytic acid combines with calcium which makes some of the calcium in legumes unavailable to meet your needs. The old method of soaking beans for 24 hours changes the phytate and decreases its action. Once again the old method of doing things is proven to be based on observation of cause and effect. The new quick method of cooking dried beans will save you time but not nutrients.

Cooked fresh legumes are a good source of vitamin A, and retain some even when dried. The fresh, cooked ones are also a good source of vitamin C, but there is none in the dried ones. But when the dried ones are left in water until they sprout, as is familiar with soybeans, the sprouts are an excellent source of vitamin C. Legumes are fair sources of the B vitamins, B_6, folacin, and pantothenic acid. Legumes are lacking in vitamin B_{12}.

Vegans and Vegetarianism

Completely vegetarian diets, though they can be made adequate in protein by careful planning and computer addition of the essential amino acid contents of the foods that complement each other's amino acid pattern, will always be deficient in vitamin B_{12}. The protein also may not be of sufficient amount and quality for the high needs of pregnancy and the growing child. Completely vegetarian diets are very bulky. For a non-pregnant woman to get the 46 grams of good-quality protein she needs each day from legumes and cereals, she would have to eat 3 cups of cooked beans plus a considerable amount of nuts, cereals, seeds, and other vegetables.

If you wish to follow a vegetarian way of eating you will be much wiser and better nourished to use eggs and milk with the plant foods. The carefully planned lacto-ovo vegetarian diet can be complete in all nutrients in adequate amounts if enough of the foods are eaten.

If you wish, or have been advised, to lower your fat intake, then using legumes as a protein source for some meals each week is one way of doing it.

Soybean

The soybean is different from other legumes. It is a protein, carbohydrate, and fat food like milk, and its protein has a biological value almost as high as meat. Its protein contains all the essential amino acids. The soybean has been the milk and steak of China for centuries. In recent years its use on this continent has been on the increase.

Soybean, as a dried bean, requires long cooking to remove its somewhat bitter taste, to make the carbohydrate more digestible, and to eliminate the antitrypsin toxin that affects protein digestion. In other words the soybean is a more useful food when it has been somewhat processed. For centuries, the Chinese and Japanese have been processing soybeans by fermentation, among other methods. From the fermented soybeans they derive such products as soya milk, which can be made into soya curd (bean curd or tofu), a common ingredient in Chinese and Japanese recipes.

In this country the soybean is processed in other ways. The beans are cleaned, cracked, hulled, and crushed into flakes. The flakes are then treated, to remove all the oil, and ground into soy grits or soy flour, which are about 50 percent protein. These products are used in baked goods, meat products, and cereals. The flakes may be further treated to remove the soluble carbohydrate and produce a soy protein concentrate that is about 67 percent protein. This high-protein supplement has been approved for use in lunches served in schools. One use of hydrated soy protein is to add half a pound of it to 1½ pounds of ground beef, which will make six burgers. These are adequate servings with a protein value of meat at a lower cost.

By further separating the soy protein from the remaining components of the concentrate, a soy protein that is 90 percent isolated is obtained. This is used in many "convenience" foods, such as sausages, coffee whiteners, frozen desserts, sour cream dips, and snack foods. These forms of soy protein are used to make textured vegetable protein (which is either extruded or spun) for use in fabricated foods.

9.
Fruits and Vegetables

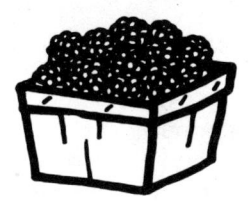

FRUITS

From the familiar "visions of sugar plums" at Christmas to the apple of the Garden of Eden, fruits are written of as foods to be enjoyed. They are the only group of foods found in nature that satisfy our sweet tooth and they have been eaten since the dawn of history. Many of our familiar fruits came from the Orient, moving first to India and then to the Mediterranean as trade routes were established. Apricots, bananas, plums, peaches, pears, and oranges all have origins in the Far East. From the Middle East come figs and dates, once called the candy that grows on trees.

Figs, dates, and grapes have a high sugar content that preserves them when they are dried—whether by desert sun or by our more modern means. By the 1400s fruits were being candied, sugared, or kept in jars in a heavy sugar syrup, and they were considered a festive treat. Grape growing expanded across Europe, mainly for the purpose of making wine, which in many areas was a safer drink than water. Since it was used when it was fairly young, it may even have had some vitamin content.

When we look at the array of fresh fruits in our present-day markets, it is hard to believe that until 1700 people died or suffered from scurvy because they did not know the cause was vitamin C deficiency and that eating an orange or lemon would protect them. Today you may face a possible lack of other nutrients, such as potassium and folacin, which are also present in citrus fruit, by using vitamin C drinks, and run the risk of deficiency of other nutrients by letting someone else, namely a food company, prepare your vegetables.

Nutrients in Fruits

Vitamin C

Fruits are one of our best sources of vitamin C, but the amount they contain varies greatly from fruit to fruit. If you check the vitamin C column in the table showing the nutritive values of fresh fruits on page 154, you may find that some have less than you thought. The citrus family is our best source of vitamin C.

Vitamin A

Fruits are among our best sources of vitamin A. The orange-colored ones, including oranges and pink grapefruits, are the best. Fruits high in vitamin A that are also high in vitamin C, such as cantaloupe and strawberries, provide a seasonal menu change but are expensive out of season.

Other Nutrients

Including fruits in your meals every day for their mineral content is as important as including them for vitamins A and C. Fruits are an excellent source of potassium, which is needed for its role in the acid-base balance of your blood and body fluids (see Chapter 4). Although there is no RDA for potassium, it is of vital importance to the overall balance of minerals for cell function and fluid control.

Some fruits have quite valuable amounts of iron, some contribute calcium, and some magnesium—further reasons to eat a wide variety of foods. Our daily requirement for B-vitamins is met by the moderate amounts supplied by many foods, and fruits also contribute some of these. In addition, fruits are one of our best sources of dietary fiber. The fiber of fruit is two forms of indigestible complex carbohydrate—pectins and cellulose.

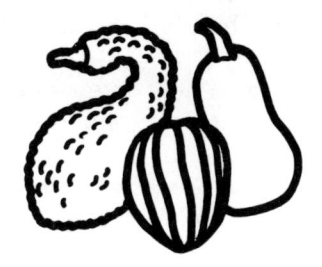

VEGETABLES

Vegetables have come to us from many lands. For example, peas came from the Orient, lettuce was popular in ancient Persia, and the cabbage family was the vitamin C vegetable of northern Europe. Potatoes, tomatoes, corn, and summer and winter squash, some of our most popular vegetables, came from the New World. It is hard to imagine Italian cooking without tomatoes, and harder yet to believe tomatoes were once considered poisonous.

Nutrients in Vegetables

Vitamin C

Vegetables are the only foods other than fruits that supply us with the vitamin C we need daily. The main difference between these two sources is that we cook most of the vegetables. The way you prepare and cook vegetables can have quite an effect on the amount of vitamin C that is lost. The following rules result in the least loss.

- Wash the vegetables well but do not let them soak in water.
- If possible, cook them in large pieces. Shredded cabbage, for instance, loses more vitamin C in cooking than cabbage wedges.
- Don't add any soda to the water.
- Cook them in as small an amount of water as possible, in a covered saucepan, just until tender. And cook them as close to serving time as possible. Quick cooking in a pressure cooker causes the least loss of vitamins.

Keeping vegetables warm and reheating them are very destructive of their vitamin C content. You must keep this in mind when using canned and especially frozen products. By their very nature, they are reheated foods and will have less vitamin C in them when eaten than the amount given on the label.

A freshly baked or even boiled potato is a good source of vitamin C. Potatoes supplied the vitamin C for many people in the days before we had orange juice so readily available. "Convenience" potato products do not have the vitamin C value of fresh potatoes, and in recent studies, frozen French-fried potatoes stored at fluctuating temperatures (between 9° and minus 10° F) lost considerable vitamin C in three months.

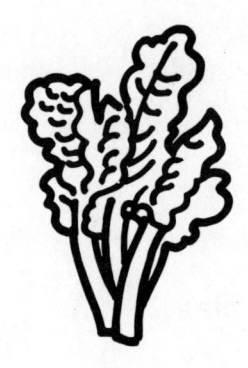

Vitamin A

While cooking vegetables causes a loss of vitamin C, it makes vitamin A more available to you. Because cooking softens the fiber and makes starches more digestible, vitamin A and the minerals are more available for absorption during the digestive processes. You may get more vitamin A from cooked carrots and leafy green vegetables than from raw. The more tender salad greens eaten raw are good sources of both vitamins A and C. Serving cooked vegetables with butter or margarine, and salads with oil, improves the absorption of the fat-soluble vitamin A.

Iron

Some vegetables are high in iron. We now know that when your body needs iron, more is absorbed from the foods you eat including vegetables. The understanding that body need regulates absorption explains why certain older studies showed that iron from vegetables was not well used while others showed that it was. Iron from food is better absorbed when vitamin C is also present, as it usually is in the iron-rich vegetables. Interestingly, some peoples of Africa consider leafy green vegetables food for children and women, who, in fact, have higher iron needs than men.

Calcium

Some vegetables, especially the leafy green ones, are high in calcium. The spinach family also has a high oxalic acid content. Since the oxalic acid combines with the calcium and our digestive systems cannot separate them, the calcium is lost. However, the calcium of vegetables that do not contain oxalic acid is well used.

Protein

Vegetables other than legumes are not concentrated sources of protein, but many have amounts that count toward your daily need. Vegetable proteins are incomplete, but if vegetables are eaten in a meal that contains complete protein, the biological value of the protein in the vegetable is increased. Protein can be made more complete if the vegetable is served with a cheese sauce or a sprinkling of cheese, toasted almonds, or peanuts.

Other Nutrients

Vegetables contribute nutrients right across the board, some in small amounts and some in considerable amounts including the trace minerals, which you can read about in Chapter 5. If you broaden your vegetable perspective, you may increase your nutrient intake.

Like fruits, vegetables are one of our best sources of indigestible carbohydrate, or fiber. It is not necessary to get fiber only from bran. Lettuce, one of our most popular vegetables, and other leafy green vegetables supply us with both folacin and fiber.

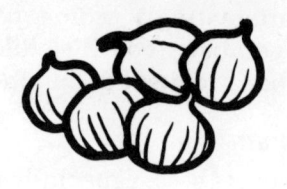

FRESH PRODUCE

Storage

All growers wish to send their produce to market in prime condition. They have been so successful in this and in lengthening the time many fruits and vegetables are available, that the present-day consumer expects to be able to buy produce year-round. On the other hand, the practices that make this possible are sometimes questioned.

Most vegetables are kept in simple cold storage. Vegetables age but do not ripen after harvesting. Some fruits are also kept in simple cold storage, with the temperature just above freezing. Others are kept in controlled-atmosphere cold storage. Fresh fruits continue to live and breathe after harvest. If this process can be slowed down, the continued ripening and eventual decomposition of the fruit can be brought almost to a standstill. This is done by keeping the fruit in an atmosphere of decreased oxygen and increased carbon dioxide.

Different fruits keep better in different atmospheres and at different temperatures. The fruit is kept in airtight rooms in a cold circulating atmosphere best for it. The storage life of apples, pears, peaches, grapes, strawberries, bananas, and oranges has been lengthened by this method. In the future, fruits may be shipped as well as stored in controlled atmospheres. This would enable the grower to let the fruits ripen more before picking them. Present-day fruits continue to ripen during transport and at the point of sale; some also require ripening after purchase.

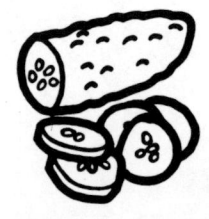

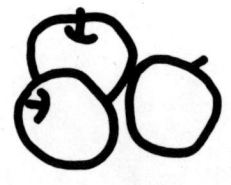

Waxing

Fruit trees and vegetable-bearing plants are sprayed by the grower with insecticides so fruits or vegetables don't get nibbled at and become homes for insects. When the fruits and vegetables are harvested, they are thoroughly washed. This removes the dirt, dust, any insecticide residue and also nature's protective coating. In nature, plants have a thin layer of wax or oil on their leaves, stems, flowers, and fruits to prevent loss of moisture. To replace nature's wax, fruits and vegetables are then sprayed either with a "food grade" paraffin, which has to have the approval of the FDA, or a wax made from palm frond.

Vegetables treated this way include cucumbers, green peppers, tomatoes, rutabagas, and sweet potatoes. Apples, citrus fruits, and melons are the fruits commonly waxed. The wax is safe and you can eat it if you wish, but all fruits should be washed before using, and the wax can be washed off. If you peel the fruit, the wax goes with the peel. If these foods were not treated this way, they would shrivel and lose quality. Some would be on the market only when in season locally.

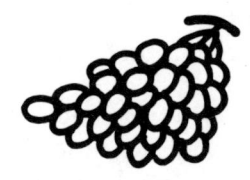

NUTRIENT CONTENT OF PROCESSED FRUITS AND VEGETABLES

Canned Fruits and Vegetables

The nutritional value of canned fruits and vegetables, as they come from the can, is almost the same as the cooked fresh fruit or vegetable. Many consumers feel that the syrup used in some canned fruits is too high in sugar. However, sugar is a preservative as well as a sweetener, and syrups may keep the shape and flavor of the fruit better than plain water does. Canners are now using lightly sweetened syrups and fruit juices to meet the needs and tastes of many consumers. By comparing the carbohydrate content of a serving of the fresh fruit, as listed in the nutrient table on page 154, with that declared on the label of the canned fruit, you can determine which comes from the fruit and which from the syrup.

In canning vegetables, salt is added to the water as the preservative. A small amount of salt is used, as in home cooking, to give the vegetables a better flavor. As it happens, water-soluble vitamins dissolve less in slightly salted water. Nevertheless, the loss of vitamin C in the liquid of canned vegetables can be considerable. The liquid can sometimes be added to homemade soups if the flavor is pleasing. The salt and flavor usually make it unsuitable for diluting canned condensed soups.

Quick-Frozen Fruits and Vegetables

The first quick-frozen vegetables came on the market in 1931. Since that time, the word *quick*, which describes an essential part of the process, has been dropped from common usage, and now consumers assume that they can freeze almost anything in the storage-freezer of their refrigerators and that it will be just as good a few weeks later. It may not have lost flavor, but in all likelihood it will have lost some vitamin content. (Of course consumers who have proper freezers and use proper methods can home-freeze foods with fairly good results.)

When vegetables are quick-frozen by industry they are picked at the right degree of maturity and taken to a nearby freezing plant. Inedible material is removed, and the vegetable is blanched by steam or boiling water. The blanching process inactivates the enzymes that cause the vegetable to continue to age and toughen. The process also inactivates an enzyme that destroys vitamin C.

The food is packed in moisture-proof and vaporproof containers and frozen at about minus 30° F (minus 35° C) so that the product is completely frozen in 30 minutes or a little longer. Vegetables such as peas and cut green beans are spread on a perforated belt that carries them through a tunnel, where they are frozen very quickly by blasts of below-zero air.

In the freezing process, the destructive enzymes are only inactivated. The colder the storage the less likelihood that any of the enzymes will become active and lower the quality of the product and destroy the vitamin C. Vitamin C and thiamin losses can be greater in frozen products than in canned.

Fruits are not as successful products when frozen, except the citrus juices. There are not many frozen fruits. They probably suffer less vitamin C loss than vegetables because the fruit acids protect the vitamin. Fruits do not contribute a great deal of thiamin, but their vitamin C is valuable. Both the time and the temperature of storage affect the losses. The longer the period of storage and the higher the temperature, the greater the losses. Some fruits may have ascorbic acid added to prevent them from darkening or turning brown. This increases their total ascorbic acid or vitamin C content and helps counteract losses.

Degrees of Temperature		Probable Loss of Vitamin C
Fahrenheit	Centigrade	
+10	−12	50% in 4 months
0	−20	50% in 8 months
−20	−30	None in 12 months

Recent studies have shown that vegetables and meats kept at temperatures that go up and down let the enzymes develop enough to cause vitamin and quality losses. These losses become important if you use frozen produce all or most of the time, especially if you are counting on them to supply the vitamin C and thiamin you expect them to have. For example freshly baked, boiled, or mashed potatoes have been constant and quite good sources of vitamin C for over two centuries. Although in the United States 10 pounds more per person were consumed in 1970 than in 1960, the amount prepared fresh dropped by 15 pounds which made a 25 pound gain in processed potatoes, most of which were frozen.

In 1976, 3.3 billion pounds of frozen potato products were used. Last year almost 2 billion pounds were sold as French-fried potatoes, 80 percent of which were served outside the home. Considering vitamin loss, it makes the potato a different food—a high-fat, low-vitamin counterpart of a once reliable, cheap source of vitamin C. The prediction is that the trend will continue. Nutritionists hope it will not.

The losses of the more recently known B-vitamins, folacin, and vitamin B_6 have not yet been analyzed.

Vitamin Loss in Three Months

	Degrees Fahrenheit	Constant Temperature	Fluctuating Temperature (20° Fluctuation)
Vitamin C			
	0	50%	72% (at +9 to −10 degrees F.)
	−4	22%	44%
	−20	almost none	31%
Thiamin	+12	7%	40%
	−4	3%	30%

CONSUMER PROTECTION

Household Storage Tips

The frozen-food industry has a Code of Recommended Practices for the handling of all frozen foods based on 0°F (−20°C). This applies to warehouses, transportation, delivery to retail stores, and storage within the stores. Consumers too should keep frozen foods at below-zero temperatures. Here are some recommendations:

- If your refrigerator has only an ice-cube section, it may only be as cold as 15 or even 20 degrees F. Some frozen foods begin to thaw at this temperature even though they are still hard. Use them within four or five days.
- If your refrigerator has one door but inside has a frozen-food compartment, it will be about 10 to 15 degrees F. If it is colder, the refrigerated foods will freeze. Frozen foods kept in such a compartment should be used in a few weeks. If you "slow-freeze" any leftovers or other cooked dishes, they will suffer losses by your processing and should be used soon.
- If your refrigerator is a "twin," with a separate freezer and refrigerator, the freezer unit will be at zero or even minus 10 degrees F, and it will keep your food for several months. If it is a self-defrost machine, the temperature should not go above zero in the defrost phase.
- If you have a separate freezer, you should not keep it higher than zero—better at minus 10 degrees F. You can then keep a wide selection at good nutritional quality for up to 12 months.

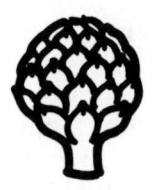

Grades of Fresh Produce

The first federal food grades were established in 1917, although over the years the various states established their own grading regulations. In 1946 the first USDA grading and inspection procedures were established at the request of the food industry. In 1953 the Agricultural Marketing Service was established, and grading was placed under its jurisdiction. But in 1977 the food-grading functions were shifted to the USDA's Food Safety and Quality Service.

According to a standard established by the Department, fresh vegetables and fruits are graded on appearance, condition, eating quality, and waste. One change that will result from the 1977 move is a uniform nomenclature for grades of fresh vegetables and fruits. The new grades are based on almost the same features as the original ones: color, size, shape, maturity, and number of defects. The differences are not nutritional, but relate to appearance and flavor. *U.S. No. 1* means good quality and is the chief grade for most fruits and vegetables. *U.S. No. 2* is the next grade, and such produce probably would not be marketed fresh.

You may not always see the grade on fresh produce because it is stamped on the shipping container. However, some packaged produce is marked with the grade. If the package has a grade shield, it means it was packed under government supervision.

Grades of Canned and Frozen Fruits and Vegetables

The grading and inspection of canned and frozen fruits and vegetables is voluntary and paid for by the producing company. Some companies have their own standards which may be even more exacting than those of the USDA. Producers of nationally advertised products spend considerable effort to maintain the same quality year after year. Unadvertised brands may also maintain a high quality and are worth getting to know since they are often lower in price. Chain stores may have their own "private" labels which meet their own standards of quality.

They may even offer two grades to their customers, one more economically priced. But whatever grade is claimed, the product must measure up.

The grades for canned and frozen fruits are given by letters and/or description rather than by numbers. *U.S. Grade A or Fancy* are vegetables and fruits with the best color. They are young or tender and free from blemishes. *U.S. Grade B or Extra Standard* are good quality, but slightly more mature and less tender. *U.S. Grade C or Standard* are not as uniform in color and flavor and are more mature than Grade B. This grade is less expensive and not all stores carry it.

The USDA has also established grades for many frozen vegetables based on flavor, color, tenderness, texture, uniformity, and absence of defects. The grades are A (Fancy), B (Extra Standard), C (Standard), and D (Substandard). As in the case of canned fruits and vegetables, some companies have more exacting standards for grading their products than the minimum allowed by the Department's grade. All frozen vegetables come under the regulations of the Food, Drug, and Cosmetic Act of 1938 and the Fair Packaging and Labeling Act of 1966.

FDA Regulations for Canned Fruits and Vegetables

The first pure food law was passed in 1906, and the first official food-grade standard, established in 1917, was for potatoes. Both have been added to and undergone many changes in order to assure us of a safe food supply. The Food, Drug and Cosmetic Act of 1938 and the Fair Packaging and Labeling Act of 1966 are the basic federal laws that apply to all foods. The two Acts and the regulations issued under them assure us that our foods are safe, wholesome, and nutritious and that they are labeled truthfully and packaged so that we cannot be deceived. The 1938 Act is for both safety and labeling and has been amended 30 times to add new regulations and modify others. The 1966 Act requires complete information on the label as to contents and packer.

Standards for Canned Fruits and Vegetables

In addition to grades, "standards" have been established for many canned fruits and vegetables.

1. A standard of identity spells out how a product must be made in order for it to be sold legally by the name on the label.

2. The quality standard: requires that the food be the quality or grade claimed on the label. The canning liquid must also meet a standard for canned fruit, and the amount of salt is specified for vegetables.
3. The standard for fill of container is specified. For example, for canned apricots the regulation requires "the maximum quantity of apricots (whole or halves) that can be sealed in the container . . . without crushing or breaking the apricots." Regulations require that the can be as full as is practicable. (Although some consumers might like the drained weight to be given, this is not possible because of differences in the shape and shrinkage of fruits when they are processed.)
4. The standard for the syrup is spelled out. There are allowable variations from slightly sweetened water to extra heavy syrup. Whatever the variation, the syrup must be of the concentration that is stated on the label. Some fruits are canned in fruit juices which are given in the ingredient listing.
5. The water used in canned foods, the pure drinking water of the place where the cannery is located, is retreated to remove undesirable chemicals and to make certain it is safe. It is called potable water.
6. Additional ingredients: The label must state if any allowed optional ingredients, such as apricot kernels, spices, or fruit juices, have been added.

Nutritional Labeling Information

Nutritional information is optional and may or may not be on the label. Some key nutrients are affected by canning. In canned fruits, vitamin A is not affected. But water-soluble vitamin C, the B-group, and certain minerals are dissolved from the fruit into the syrup. The heavier the syrup, the less are dissolved; but if the syrup is eaten with the fruit, the vitamins and minerals are not actually lost.

You can compare information on the label with the nutrient value of fresh produce in the Table, page 154. There are further losses of vitamin C and thiamin between the time a fruit is canned and the time you use it; 10 to 25 percent is lost during a year, the smaller losses being in products kept in cool storage. If the canned fruit is used in cooked dessert, there are additional losses.

In canned vegetables, vitamin A is not affected a great deal by the canning process, but water-soluble vitamin C and the B-vitamins are lost in the liquid. The greatest loss is of thiamin, which is also affected by the heat processing. There are additional losses when you heat the vegetables.

NUTRITIVE VALUE OF FRESH FRUIT AS EATEN RAW

	Amount	Energy Calories (gm)	Carbo-hydrate (gm)	Protein (gm)	Calcium (mg)	Phosphorus (mg)	Magnesium (mg)	Sodium (mg)	Potassium (mg)
Apples—2½ inch	1	58	15		7	10	8	1	100
Apricots, medium	3	51	13	1	17	23	12	1	281
Banana, medium	1	127	34	2	12	39	50	1.5	555
Blackberries, Boysenberries, Youngberries	⅔ c	58	13	1	32	19	30	1	170
Blueberries	⅔ c	62	15	1	15	13	6		81
Cherries, red sour, pitted	⅔ c	58	14	1	22	19	—	2	191
Cherries, sweet	14	70	17	1	22	19	14	2	191
Cranberries, chopped	¼ c	12	3		3	2	—	.5	20
Cranberry-orange relish, raw	¼ c	120	31		13	5	—	.7	
Dates	12	274	73	2	59	63	58	1	648
Figs, fresh, medium	2	80	20	1	35	22	20	2	195
Grapefruit, seedless, pink	½ med	40	10		16	16	12	1	138
white	½ med	40	10		16	16	12	1	135
Grapes, seedless	20	67	17		12	20	13	3	173
Guava, common	3½ oz	62	15		23	42	—	4	289
Kumquats	1 med	13	3		12	4	—	1.4	47
Lemon juice	½ c	25	8		7	10	8	3	141
Mango	⅔ c	66	17		10	13	—	7	189
Melons, Canteloupe balls	⅔ c	30	8		14	16	16	12	251
Honeydew balls	⅔ c	33	8		14	16	—	12	251
Watermelon balls	⅔ c	26	6		7	10	8	1	100
Nectarine	1 large	96	25		6	36	20	9	441
Orange—3 inch	1	75	18	1	61	30	16	1.5	300
Orange juice	¾ c	80	19	1	20	30	19	1.8	381
Papaya, cubes	¾ c	39	10		20	16	+	3	234
Peaches, peeled, 2½ inch	1	38	10		9	19	10	1	202
Pear, Bartlett, 3-inch	1	109	28	1	14	20	13	3.0	234
Persimmon	½	65	16		5	22	8	3	174
Pineapple, cubes	⅔ c	52	14		17	8	13	1	146
Plums, prune, fresh (medium)	3	75	20		12	18	9	1	170
Prunes, dried, softenized (med)	4	80	22		16	25	13	2	224
Raisins (snack package)	½ oz	45	12		9	14	5	4	114
Rhubarb, cooked with sugar	½ c	190	49		105	20	13	2.7	274
Strawberries	⅔ c	37	8		21	21	12	1	164

\+ Probably present.
— No data.
Blank space—insignificant.

Iron mg	Zinc mg	Vitamin A IU	Vitamin C mg	Thiamin mg	Riboflavin mg	Niacin mg	Vitamin B₆ mg	Pantothenic Acid mg	Folacin mcg
.3	.05	90	4	.03	.02	.1	.03	.11	8
.5	—	2700	10	.03	.04	.6	.07	.24	3
1.1	.04	285	15	.07	.09	1.0	.76	.39	42
.9	—	200	21	.03	.04	.4	.05	.24	14
1.0	—	100	14	.03	.06	.5	.07	.16	8
.4	—	1000	10	.05	.06	.4			
.4	—	110	10	.05	.06	.4	.03	.26	8
.1	—	10	3					1	
.3	—	46	12	.02	.01	—	—		1
3.0	—	50	0	.09	.10	2.2	.15	.78	21
.6	—	80	2	.06	.05	.4	.11	.30	9
.4	.10	440	37	.04	.02	.2	.03	.28	11
.4	.10	10	37	.04	.02	.2	.03	.28	11
.4	—	100	4	.05	.03	.3	.08	.07	7
.9	—	280	242	.05	.05	.1	—		—
.1	—	120	7	.02	.02	—	—		—
.2	—	20	46	.03	.01	.1	.05	.10	12
.4	—	4800	35	.05	.05	1.1	—		—
.4	—	3400	33	.04	.03	.6	.09	.25	30
.4	—	40	23	.04	.03	6	.06	.20	+
.5	—	590	7	.03	.03	.2	.07	.30	8
.8	—	2475	20	+	+	+	.03	+	30
.6	.15	300	75	.15	.06	.7	.09	.36	65
.4	.04	370	83	.17	.06	.7	.09	.33	102
.3	—	1750	56	.04	.04	.3	+	.22	+
.5	.20	1330	7	.02	.05	1.0	.03	.17	8
.5	.46	36	7	.03	.07	.2	.03	.13	25
.2	—	2275	9	.03	.01	.1	.01		
.5	.15	70	17	.09	.03	.2	.09	.16	11
.5	—	1340	4	.03	.03	.5	.05	.19	6
1.2	—	510	1	.03	.05	.5	.08	.15	2
.5	—	2	+	.01	.01	.1	.03	.01	1
.8	—	110	8	.03	.07	.4	.03	.07	9
1.0	.08	60	59	.03	.07	.6	.06	.34	16

NUTRITIVE VALUE OF FRESH VEGETABLES AS EATEN COOKED UNLESS NOTED "RAW."

	Amount	Weight gm	Energy Calories	Carbo-hydrate gm	Protein gm	Calcium mg	Phosphorus mg	Magnesium mg	Sodium mg
Artichoke, globe (100 gm edible)	1	160	52	10	3	51	69	—	30
Asparagus	6 spears	100	20	4	2	21	50	20	1
Avocado, raw	½	100	171	6	2	10	42	45	4
Beans, green	¾ c	100	25	5	2	50	37	32	4
Bean sprouts	⅔ c	60	28	5	3	17	48	—	4
Beets	½ c	85	27	6	1	12	20	23	36
Broccoli	⅔ c	100	26	5	3	88	62	24	10
Brussels sprouts	6 or 7	100	36	6	4	32	72	—	10
Cabbage, shredded	⅔ c	100	20	4	1	44	20	—	14
shredded, raw	½ c	50	12	3	1	25	15	6	10
Carrots,	⅔ c	100	31	7	1	33	31	—	33
grated, raw	½ c	50+	21	5	—	18	18	13	24
Cauliflower	¾ c	100	22	4	2	21	42	—	9
Celery, sliced	¾ c	100	14	3	1	31	22	—	88
raw, 5×¾"	3 pieces	50	8	2	—	20	14	11	63
Chard, Swiss	½ c	100	18	3	2	73	24	65	86
Collards	½ c	100	33	5	4	188	52	57	—
Corn, sweet kernels	½ c	100	83	19	3	3	89	48	—
Cucumber, raw	6 slices	25	4	1	—	4	5	3	1
Eggplant	2 slices	100	19	4	1	11	21	16	1
Endive, escarole (raw)	1 c	50	10	2	—	41	27	5	7
Kale	½ c	50	20	3	3	93	29	18*	22
Lettuce, iceberg (raw)	⅙ head	90	12	3	1	18	20	10	8
Bibb, romaine (raw)	1 c	50	9	2	1	34	13	—	4
Mushrooms, raw	½ c	35	9	1	1	2	39	3	5
Mustard greens	⅔ c	100	23	4	2	138	32	27	18
Onions, boiled	½ c	100	29	7	1	24	29	—	7
Parsnips	⅔ c	100	66	15	1	45	62	32	8
Peas, green	⅔ c	100	71	12	5	23	99	35	1
Pepper, green, sweet	1 med	100	18	4	1	9	16	12	9
raw	¼ c	25	6	1	+	2	6	5	3
Pimiento (red, sweet) canned	1 pod	40	10	2	+	3	+	—	—
Potato, baked	1 med	150	140	31	4	13	98	33	6
Pumpkin, canned	1 c	245	80	19	2	61	64	30	49
Rutabaga	½ c	125	43	10	1	75	39	19	5
Spinach	½ c	90	20	3	3	84	34	—	45
raw	1 c	50	13	2	1	47	25	44	35
Squash, summer, all (cubes)	½ c	100	14	3	1	25	25	16	1
winter, all (mashed)	½ c	100	38	9	1	20	32	17	1
Sweet potato, baked	1 med	150	211	48	3	60	87	46	18
Tomato,	½ c	120	32	7	2	18	38	15	4
raw	1 med	150	32	7	2	19	40	21	4
juice	¾ c	180	35	8	2	13	32	18	360

NOTE: ½ Avocado contains 17 gm fat.
* Figure for raw vegetable.

+ Probably present.
— No data.

Potassium (mg)	Iron (mg)	Zinc (mg)	Vitamin A (IU)	Vitamin C (mg)	Thiamin (mg)	Riboflavin (mg)	Niacin (mg)	Vitamin B-6 (mg)	Pantothenic Acid (mg)	Folacin (mcg)
301	1.1	—	150	8	.07	.04	.7	—	—	—
183	.6	—	900	26	.16	.18	1.4	.06	.20	109
604	.6	2.4	290	14	.11	.20	1.6	.42	1.07	51
151	.6	.3	540	12	.07	.09	.5	.08	.19	40
156	.9	—	20	6	.09	.10	.7	—	—	145
177	.4	.4	17	5	.03	.03	.3	.05	.13	66
267	.8	.2	2500	90	.09	.20	.8	.19	1.17	56
273	1.1	—	520	87	.08	.14	.8	—	—	36
163	.3	.4	130	33	.04	.04	.3	—	—	18
116	.2	.2	65	26	.03	.03	.2	.08	.10	33
222	.6	.3	10500	6	.05	.05	.5	—	—	24
170	.4	.2	5500	4	.03	.03	.3	.08	.12	18
206	.7	—	60	55	.09	.08	.6	—	—	34
239	.2	—	230	6	.02	.03	.3	—	—	—
170	.2	—	120	5	.01	.01	.2	.03	.22	6
321	1.8	—	5400	16	.04	.11	.4	—	.17	42
262	.8	.7	7800	76	.11	.20	1.2	.20	.50	102*
165	.6	.3	400	7	.11	.10	1.3	.20	.22	33*
40	.1	+	+	3	+	.01	+	.01	.06	4
150	.6	—	10	3	.05	.04	.5	—	—	16
147	.8	—	1650	5	.03	.07	.3	.01	.05	26
110	.8	—	4150	45	.05	.09	.8	.09	.18	30*
157	.5	.4	297	5	.05	.05	.3	.05	.18	37
132	.7	—	950	9	.03	.04	.2	—	—	90
138	.3	.1	—	1	.03	.15	1.4	.04	.73	8
220	1.8	.2	5800	48	.08	.14	.6	.13	.16	60
110	.4	.3	40	7	.03	.03	.2	.06*	.06*	10
379	.6	—	30	10	.07	.08	.1	.09	.60	23
196	1.8	.7	540	20	.28	.11	2.3	.05	.15	25
149	.5	.1	420	96	.06	.07	.5	—	—	—
53	—	—	105	32	.02	.02	.1	.07	.06	5
109	.6	—	920	38	.01	.02	.2	—	—	—
753	1	.5	+	30	.15	.06	2.5	.35	.6	26
588	1	+	15680	12	.07	.12	1.5	.14	.98	47
207	.4	—	688	33	.07	.07	1.0	.13	.20	26
291	2	.6	7290	25	.06	.12	.5	.12	.07	82
235	1.6	.5	4050	25	.05	.10	.3	.14	.15	106
141	.4	.4	390	10	.05	.08	.8	.06	.17	11
258	.5	—	3500	8	.04	.10	.4	.09	.28	12
450	1.3	—	12150	33	.13	.11	1	.33	1.2	26
344	.8	.2	1200	29	.08	.06	1	.11	.3	32
366	.7	.3	1350	35	.09	.06	1	.15	.48	59
409	1.6	.3	1460	29	.09	.05	1.5	.35	.45	47

10.
Foods from Grains

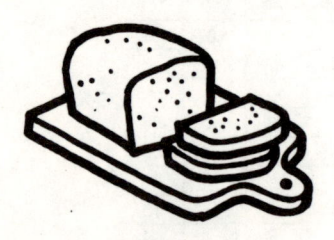

Cereal grains and the foods made from them have been the main source of energy and one of the main sources of protein for mankind since man first learned how to grow food. The early Egyptians started wheat culture that provided enough food for even the poorest people, thus freeing them for work other than seeking food. Similarly, rice was the protein-calorie food that enabled the peoples of the Orient to develop their highly civilized cultures. The word "rice" means "agriculture" in the Chinese language. Half the world's population depend on rice as their main source of food.

Barley, grown as early as wheat and rice, was a staple food of the Greeks, Romans, Egyptians, and Chinese. Although we use little barley today, it was the chief grain for making bread in Europe as late as the 1500s. Oats, which we use more than barley, were cultivated later than the other grains, and then mostly in northern Europe. From early days, oats have been grown as a feed grain for animals.

Rye is another grain of northern Europe. It makes a very heavy bread unless mixed with part wheat flour, as our rye breads are. It too is grown as a feed grain. Corn, an American grain, was the staple food for ancient Mexican and Central American peoples, as it is still today.

NUTRITIVE CONTENT

From the very beginning of their use as food, the cereal grains have been cooked. Uncooked or raw mature dried grain is a hard seed, very difficult for us to digest. The cooking methods we use today are little different from those used in earliest times. The ancient people of the Near East combined wheat with a fairly large quantity of water in an iron kettle and cooked it over a low fire. The ancient Orientals cooked their rice the same way, over a small charcoal fire much as they do today.

Water softens the outside bran coating, loosening it. The inside cells of starch absorb the water, swell up and burst. Both the starch and the protein that formed the cell are made more digestible by the process.

The cooked starch is said to be *hydrolysed*, which is a term often seen in the list of ingredients of "convenience" foods. The cooked grain is from three to four times the volume of the uncooked. If the grain is cooked in the right amount of water, so all is absorbed, no water-soluble minerals and vitamins are lost.

Of all the grains, raw rice is the least changed by the way we use it. Brown rice contains the germ and can thus become rancid unless kept refrigerated. Enriched white rice has added vitamins sprayed on the surface of the clean grain. Follow the package directions for cooking rice. Rice that is parboiled has been steamed before the bran is removed. By this method of removing the bran some of the vitamins in the bran are absorbed by the carbohydrate center of the kernel. If the bran is polished off, there is more vitamin loss.

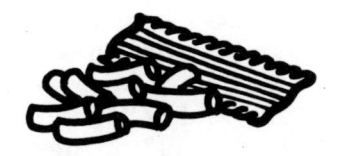

PROTEIN

In our calorie-counting society, we have tended to downgrade the grain foods because they are concentrated sources of energy. This is unfortunate because they can supply us with a good amount of protein without any accompanying fat.

The proteins of cereals have also been downgraded. Cereal proteins do not have all of the essential amino acids, but food containing the missing ones, when eaten at the same time, can make up the difference. It doesn't matter to your body where the amino acids come from, as long as all that are necessary are present in your bloodstream at the same time. It is the total mixture, not the source, that is important. (For more on amino acids and the making of proteins see Chapter 3, page 37.)

One of the proteins of wheat is gluten, which makes it possible for ground wheat to become a workable, stretchable dough. Ground wheat can be made into pasta, unleavened and leavened bread, and all sorts of crackers, cakes, and cookies. Wheat proteins lack the amino acid lysine, but when we eat wheat products with milk, meat, fish, eggs, poultry, or legumes, the wheat protein is completely used. Wheat's highest quality protein is in the germ. Whole wheat flour is made from grinding the whole wheat kernels and is therefore higher in protein and some other nutrients than enriched white flour.

Rice cannot be used in as many ways as wheat because it does not have protein like gluten. Rice proteins lack the amino acids lysine and threonine. When we eat rice with milk, eggs, meat, fish, poultry, legumes, peanuts, and almonds, we can use the rice protein completely.

Corn also lacks a protein like gluten, so it cannot be used in as many ways as wheat, but when cornmeal is combined with wheat, it makes our familiar cornbread. The proteins of corn lack the amino acids lysine and tryptophan. As is the case with wheat and rice, when we eat corn with a complete protein food its proteins are better used. The proteins of corn can also be improved by eating corn with legumes, as is done in Mexico.

Like the other grains, oats lack the amino acid lysine but are quite high in protein. They are an excellent cereal when used with milk. Barley is also a high-protein grain, but it too lacks lysine. We are not great barley consumers, but in some countries barley is preferred to rice or wheat for making pilaf and for stuffing meats and poultry. When used this way or in soups containing meat, the protein is made complete. Rye is popular with us, mostly in bread. Its lack of lysine is well balanced by some combinations that are traditional in northern Europe, such as rye bread with cheese or smoked fish.

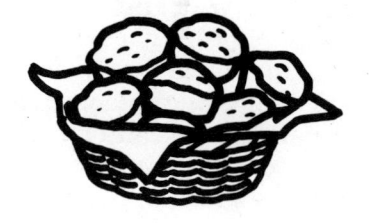

CARBOHYDRATES

The complex carbohydrates are our best source of energy, and our best and cheapest food source of complex carbohydrates are the grains. Unrefined grains are our highest sources of indigestible carbohydrates or fiber.

A Note About Potatoes

Potatoes are not a cereal but they are used in our meal patterns as a major carbohydrate food source of energy, as cereals and bread are. Countries that do not use potatoes use a great deal more grain as rice, pasta, and cracked wheat than we do. Potatoes are included in the table of grain foods at the end of this chapter, so you can compare their value with cereals. They have a similar ratio of protein to carbohydrate and supply us with a number of minerals, especially potassium. When fresh, potatoes are a good source of vitamin C also.

VITAMINS, ESPECIALLY THE B-GROUP, AND MINERALS

Since a kernel of grain is a seed containing a germ that when planted will grow into a new stalk of grain, it contains minute amounts of all the minerals the new plant will need. All grains—wheat to a greater extent than the others—contain a phosphorus compound called phytic acid. It is present in the bran layers of the grain, and because it combines with some of the calcium and iron of the grain, these minerals may not be well absorbed during digestion. Even with this disadvantage, grains are a good source of iron. If you combine them with milk, as in cereals and baked products, the milk calcium balances the calcium lost from the grain.

Whole grains are a fair source of zinc—oats, hard wheat, and wheat germ are better than corn and rice. Whole wheat is a good source of magnesium. In addition to providing thiamin and niacin, whole grains are good sources of vitamin B_6, pantothenic acid, and folacin, and some riboflavin. The germ or small part at one end of each kernel that sprouts into a new plant, is both high in fat and one of our best sources of vitamin E. The only grain that gives us any vitamin A is yellow corn. None of the grains contains any vitamin C.

Different parts of the grain kernel contain different amounts of the various nutrients. (See the table of wheat values in the next section.)

LOSS OF NUTRIENTS FROM REFINING AND MILLING

All the grain we use for food is refined to some extent. Probably corn on the cob is the only one we simply husk, cook, and eat. Other grains have a very tough outside cover on each kernel. When this husk is removed, you are left with the grain—whole wheat, brown rice, whole corn, oats, and so forth. Ground fresh grain does not keep. The oil in the germ becomes rancid. When the germ is eliminated, the ground grain or flour keeps much better. When you buy raw wheat germ, it should be refrigerated, both where you buy it and at home. Some wheat-germ products are treated to prevent the fat from becoming rancid.

When wheat is refined today, the germ and additional outside layers of each kernel are removed until all the brown bran is off and the kernel is white. This is done because (1) the flour will keep and not change in flavor or quality from the time it is milled to the time it is used: (2) refined wheat is more completely digested; and (3) refined white flour produces baked products of finer texture and appeal. It became apparent in the 1940's, as knowledge of the B-vitamins increased, that the advantages of milling were less desirable because a lot of food value is lost. The table below shows how the nutrients are divided in wheat.

PERCENTAGE OF NUTRIENTS IN A KERNEL OF WHEAT

	White Inside (83%)	Bran (14%)	Wheat Germ (2½%)*
Protein	70–75%	19%	8%
Thiamin (B$_1$)	3%	33%	64%
Riboflavin	32%	42%	26%
Niacin	12%	86%	2%
Pyridoxine (B$_6$)	6%	73%	21%
Pantothenic acid	43%	50%	7%
Vitamin E	0%	0%	100%

* The rest is lost in processing

CONSUMER PROTECTION

Enrichment

Three terms are used to describe the addition of nutrients to food products; they are most commonly seen on grain products.

> *Restored:* vitamins and minerals are returned to the food at the same level as in the original food.
> *Enriched:* vitamins and minerals that are naturally present in the food are added at levels a little higher than the natural level before processing.
> *Fortified:* vitamins, minerals, and sometimes protein that are not in the food naturally as well as nutrients naturally in the food that have been affected by processing are added.

The first enrichment regulations recommending that some of the nutrients removed in milling be returned to white flour and bread were enacted in 1941. At that time, pellagra was a tremendous health problem in the southern states, and the government made a regulation that thiamin, niacin, riboflavin, and iron be added to bread. This improved bread was given the official name "enriched" under an order from the War Food Administration and was the required bread throughout World War II. At the end of the war, enriched bread was required by law in 26 states.

Also in 1941 the breakfast cereal companies restored thiamin, niacin, and iron to the same levels as present in whole grain. In 1961 the National Research Council adopted a policy on the addition of nutrients to foods—revised in 1968 and 1973. In 1973 the enrichment of grain foods was extended to include flour, bread, white rice, degerminated cornmeal, corn grits, whole grain, and some other products. The nutrients added are thiamin, niacin, riboflavin, and iron.

Standards of Identity for Bread and Pasta

Three forms in which we use the grain foods are breads, pasta, and breakfast cereals. The FDA has established "standards of identity" for breads, rolls, pasta, and all the enriched products mentioned above. The amount of thiamin, niacin, riboflavin, and iron that is added is stated in their regulations.

Breads can be made only from allowable ingredients. If the bread label says "enriched" the bread must be made with enriched flour, which also must have a specific amount of thiamin, niacin, riboflavin, and iron. If the label says "whole wheat," the bread must be made with whole wheat flour. If the label says "raisin," the bread must be made with a certain number of ounces of raisins.

Ninety percent of our bread is enriched. In all cases, enriched bread has nutrition labeling, and the baked loaf must have the percent of the U.S. RDA for thiamin, niacin, riboflavin, calcium, iron, as well as the grams of protein, carbohydrate, and fat declared for a serving, or slice.

There are three advantages in making wheat into bread. One is the addition of calcium and milk solids to improve the texture of the dough and add to its calcium content. Another is the action of yeast in reducing the phytates that would combine with the iron, so that you get more iron when you eat a slice of bread. Also, as the yeast grows to raise the bread, it becomes a source of folacin; unleavened bread does not have this advantage.

Pasta is usually made of durum wheat, a hard wheat, which contains a lot of gluten that gives the pasta good texture and protein value. Pasta can be made of other flours, however. The kind of flours and the other ingredients allowable are regulated by the FDA code. If the flour used is enriched, the pasta will have nutrition labeling, and each pound of the pasta must contain a specific amount of thiamin, niacin, riboflavin, and iron.

Enriched pasta may also contain a specific amount of vitamin D, calcium, and wheat germ as optional ingredients.

BREAKFAST CEREALS

The breakfast cereals that are most like the original grain are the uncooked cereals that have had a minimum of processing. Cereal processing consists of steaming the grain to make it soft enough to be rolled into flakes. Each kernel becomes a flake. Regular rolled oats are rolled whole grains of oats. Quick-cooking cereals are grain kernels that are cut into three or four pieces before the steaming process and then rolled into thinner flakes. Whole-grain wheat cereals are made this way, as are quick-cooking oats. Corn grits are cut but not rolled. Instant cereals are made by special processes in which the dry grain is heated by dry heat to develop flavor before steaming.

Some "convenience" cereals are also treated with or contain alkaline salts to soften the fiber and speed the cooking. This practice is another version of the old custom of adding baking soda to vegetables to speed the cooking and prevent color change. Some vitamins are destroyed in alkaline water, so the practice is not recommended in vegetable cookery. Cereals are either enriched or fortified following this process, restoring some of the vitamin loss. These cereals are, however, often very high in sodium.

Ready-to-Eat Cereals

Each cereal company has its own methods, but in general, grains go through similar steps to be made into ready-to-eat cereals. First, the grain is cleaned. Then it is milled to various stages. Corn is a larger kernel than wheat or oats and is usually split into grits. The ingredients of the cereal are then mixed—if it consists of more than one grain and if it is flavored. The heat-stable vitamins and minerals are added at this time, and water to soften the grain. The whole mixture is then cooked like a great big batch of porridge, often using as much as a ton of grain.

Following cooking, the mixture is dried with hot air for several hours to evaporate some of the water. The softened grain is then formed in one of several ways.

- Puffed grains are softened whole kernels of rice or wheat which are shot into a vacuum where they more or less "explode."
- Flakes are made by rolling the softened grits or whole kernels under great pressure.
- Shredded cereals are forced through spinnerets and the strands are spun into biscuits.
- When a mixture of grains is used for flakes, the mixture is extruded into small pellets and then rolled into flakes.
- Some cereals are extruded into shapes such as stars, circles, letters, bubbles, etc.

After the cereal has been shaped, it is toasted by being tumbled through very hot air in ovens for a short time. This makes the cereal crisp and dry and gives it its toasted flavor. Finally, with only one or two exceptions, the cereal is fortified with the vitamins that are affected by heat. These vitamins are in a solution which is sprayed on the cereal. Some cereals are also sugared. Two of the vitamins that are added to cereals are destroyed by light. These are riboflavin and vitamin B_6. For this reason, you should not store fortified cereals in clear glass canisters.

Unsweetened and Sweetened Breakfast Cereals

Although we have reduced the incidence of deficiency diseases dramatically by the enrichment and fortification of our cereal foods, we may have opened a Pandora's box to a host of industry practices we have yet to evaluate.

In 1955 the first breakfast cereal fortified with vitamins and protein came on the market. In 1961 the first breakfast cereal fortified with 100 percent of our needs for several vitamins came on the market. From 1969 to 1976 the nutritional fortification of cereal was accelerated until more than 92 percent of our breakfast cereals were fortified with nutrients to some degree. On the whole, the restoration and fortification of milled grain products with needed nutrients has been very beneficial to the health of many people.

Moderately fortified, unsweetened, ready-to-eat cereals are good foods. When they are eaten with half a cup or more of milk, they make a fair breakfast, certainly a better one than none at all. But no group of foods has been so distorted from its original nutritional contribution than the highly presweetened and highly fortified ready-to-eat breakfast cereals. About one-third of the cereal market is for presweetened cereals.

The basic grains are excellent foods, but the presweetened or highly fortified ready-to-eat cereals are not the answer. They do not supply a balance of nutrients.

In presweetened cereals, the energy or calorie level is supplied by sugar above the level of the natural grain. Then, even if it is matched by adding certain minerals and vitamins, we need other nutrients that are not added. The use of sugar has been shown to be harmful to young, not fully calcified teeth. The addition of marshmallow candy, which is a sticky type of candy, is even more harmful. This candy, which is colored and shaped to represent dried fruit in some cereals, is a further distortion of a basic food. Even one serving of these cereals a day is a questionable amount to give to children.

Sugar has to be listed on the package along with the other ingredients, all of which are listed in order of their predominance by weight. This is confusing because our recipes usually give the volume, not the weight, of foods. When sugar is listed first its weight can be equal to or more than the weight of the cereal. For example, half an ounce of puffed wheat measures 1⅓ measuring cups, and half an ounce of sugar measures about 3½ measuring teaspoons, which is quite a bit of sugar to sprinkle on that amount of cereal. Some companies are specifying the weight of sugar added, as shown in the following table on carbohydrate information.

CARBOHYDRATE INFORMATION

1 ounce of Cereal, or 28.3 grams

Starch and related carbohydrates	15 gm (½ oz plus)
Sucrose and other sugars	11 gm (about 1 tbsp)
Total	26 gm (about 1 oz)

NUTRITIVE VALUE OF FOODS FROM GRAINS AS EATEN

	Amount	Energy Calories	Carbo-hydrate gm	Protein gm	Calcium mg	Phosphorus mg	Magnesium mg	Sodium mg	Potassium mg
Barley, cooked	¾ c	175	39	4	8	94	18	2	80
Corn, grits, enriched	⅔ c	83	18	2	3	16	7	.9	18
Corn, grits, enriched, instant	⅔ c	80	18	2	2	16	+	347	+
Cornmeal, enriched	⅔ c	82	17	2	4	43	+	.2	+
Cornmeal, degermed, enriched	⅔ c	80	18	2	2	23	17	.2	24
Oats, rolled, whole grain	⅔ c	107	18	4	14	91	40	2	98
Oats, rolled, instant	1 pkg	107	19	4	24	105	35	280	101
Rice, brown	¾ c	174	37	4	17	106	33	3	103
Rice, white, enriched	¾ c	167	38	3	16	43	15	4	43
parboiled, enriched	¾ c	139	31	3	25	75	15	3	56
instant, enriched	¾ c	135	30	3	4	23	+	338	—
Wheat, whole grain cereal	1 c	110	23	4	17	127	41	5	118
farina, enriched	1 c	100	22	3	147	127	7	.6	25
farina, quick	1 c	100	21	3	147	150	10	461	32
farina, mix & eat	1 c	100	21	3	10	38	—	235	24
Ready-to-eat Cereals									
Whole-grain, not enriched									
puffed rice, restored	1 c	60	13	1	3	14	—	—	15
puffed wheat, restored	1 c	55	12	2	4	48	—	+	51
shredded wheat biscuit	1 large	90	20	2	11	97	38	—	87
wheat germ, toasted	¼ c	110	13	9	12	300	80	1	227
Fortified, 25% of U.S. RDA									
flakes, corn	1 c	110	25	2	1	10	0	278	34
oat	⅔ c	110	20	5	40	100	0	315	100
wheat	¾ c	100	24	2	10	60	32	355	134
Extruded mixed grains	¾ c	110	20	4	40	—	8	200	—
Vitamin & Iron Supplement Cereals									
+ Protein + 50% of U.S. RDA	⅓ c	110	15	12	14	60	16	127	36
+ 100% of U.S. RDA for Vitamins	¾ c	110	24	3	40	40	16	418	60
Wheat flour, whole grain	1 c	400	85	16	49	446	128	3	444
white enriched	1 c	420	88	12	18	100	28	2	109
Bread, white enriched	1 slice	70	13	2	21	24	6	126	26
whole wheat	1 slice	65	14	3	24	71	22	126	72
rye (⅔% rye)	1 slice	80	17	3	27	73	20	182	145
Pasta, enriched macaroni, etc.	1 c	190	39	7	14	85	36	—	103

At present there is no standard for enrichment of ready-to-eat cereals. The nutritive values vary with the company.
+ Probably present.
— No data.

Iron mg	Zinc mg	Thiamin mg	Riboflavin mg	Niacin mg	Vitamin B-6 mg	Pantothenic Acid mg	Folacin mcg	Vitamin E mg	Vitamin A IU	Vitamin B-12 mcg	Vitamin C mg	Vitamin D IU
1	+	.06	.03	1.6	.11	.25	10	—	0	0	0	0
.5	.1	.1	.05	.6	.10	0	—	—	125	0	0	0
1.3	+	.2	.12	1.6	.08	0	—	—	—	0	0	0
.6	+	.1	.06	.8	.12	0	—	—	109	0	0	0
.6	.2	.1	.06	.8	.06	.16	5	.2	100	0	0	0
1	1	.13	.03	.2	.04	.22	15	.3	—	0	0	0
1	1	.15	.04	.3	.04	—	—	—	0	0	0	0
.8	.9	.14	.03	2.0	.20	.45	30	.15	0	0	0	0
1.4	.6	.17	.02	1.6	.05	.22	18	0	0	0	0	0
1.1	.5	.14	.02	1.6	—	—	20	—	0	0	0	0
1	.3	.16	—	1.2	—	—	—	—	0	0	0	0
1.2	1.2	.15	.05	1.5	.11	.20	118	.7	—	0	0	0
.8	.2	.12	.07	1	.02	.21	43	0	0	0	0	0
8	—	.15	.08	1	—	—	—	—	0	0	0	0
8	—	.15	.08	1	—	—	—	—	0	0	0	0
.3	—	.07	.01	.7	.02	.10	6	0	0	0	0	0
.6	.7	.08	.03	1.2	.05	0	0	0	0	0	0	0
.9	.8	.06	.03	1.1	.07	.20	14	0	0	0	0	0
1.8	4.5	.45	.17	1.2	.20	.40	118	4.5	40	0	1	8
1.8	3.6	.38	.43	5	.50	0	100	0	1250	1.5	15	40
4.5	3.8	.38	.43	5	.50	0	100	0	1250	1.5	0	40
4.5	3.8	.38	.43	5	.50	0	100	0	1250	1.5	15	40
4.5	3	.38	.43	5	.50	0	0	0	1250	1.5	15	40
9	.6	.75	.85	10.0	1.0	0	200	15	2500	2	30	200
18	.3	1.50	1.70	20.0	2.0	0	400	30	5000	6	60	400
4	2.9	.66	.14	5.2	.34	1.1	65	—	0	0	0	0
3.3	.8	.74	.46	6.1	.06	.47	29	—	0	0	0	0
.6	.2	.10	.06	.8	.01	.11	10	—	0	0	0	0
.8	.5	.09	.03	.8	.04	.18	16	.11	0	0	0	0
.8	.4	.09	.07	.6	.05	.16	6	—	0	0	0	0
1.4	.7	.23	.13	1.8	.1	.3	13	—	0	0	0	0

Vitamin and Mineral Supplements

Certain cereals are so highly fortified with nutrients that they are required by a 1974 FDA regulation to be labeled "vitamin and mineral supplement." These cereals are fortified with added nutrients at levels as high as from 50 to 100 percent of the U.S. RDA. Among the many minerals and vitamins added is vitamin D. They are really a cereal form of a vitamin-mineral capsule, not a balanced breakfast food. The inclusion of vitamin D at 100 percent level is a questionable practice, as we can soon build up amounts of this vitamin that are toxic. As most cereals are eaten with milk and most of our milk has added vitamin D, even the label tells you you are getting 110% or 10% too much of the U.S. RDA. These cereals should not be used by adults, or by children or teenagers during the summer. Sunshine produces vitamin D in the skin. These supplements also should not be eaten if you take vitamin capsules containing vitamin D.

How can you tell a real cereal? Since the ingredients in a product must be declared on the label, the kind of grain will be listed along with the names of any added vitamins and minerals. A long list of ingredients indicates a "fabricated cereal." The grams of protein and carbohydrate in a cereal product should be in about the same proportion as in the pure grain. You can check against the table of composition for grain foods on page 168. The usual proportion in a 1-ounce serving of an unsweetened ready-to-eat cereal is 2 to 4 grams of protein for every 16 to 20 grams of carbohydrate. When a label states "protein: 1 gram" and "carbohydrate: 25 grams" it indicates that there is more carbohydrate, usually sugar, in the cereal than was in the original grain.

Consumer Protection

Cereals come under the pure food regulations, the ingredient listing regulations, and nutritionally labeling regulations. But no standard of identity has been established as to their composition.

11.

Food Sources of Fat

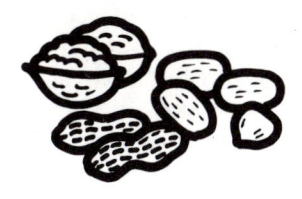

Many of the foods that we eat for protein, minerals, and vitamins also contain fat. In addition, we eat food fats and oils that contain practically no nutrients other than vitamin E. There are also high-fat foods that supply other nutrients in small amounts. If you are at least moderately active, it is all right if some high-calorie fat foods are part of your food intake. If you are not active, the amount you use should be limited.

Alcohol (in the form of gin, liqueurs, vodka, whiskies, and even wines) is very like a refined fat in that it is a source of calories without any additional nutrients. The contribution of calories per gram of alcohol makes the caloric yield closer to fat than to carbohydrate. And in the body, alcohol is metabolized less like glucose and more like fats.

HOW MUCH FAT AND WHAT KIND

Polyunsaturated and Saturated Fats

Why, how, and where our bodies use, make, and store fats is discussed in Chapter 2. The amount used by people in this country is higher than in any other country and has been going up every year. The increase has been in the consumption of polyunsaturated fats. Because of a false sense of security given by publicity and advertising, many people have the idea that if a fat is polyunsaturated, somehow it isn't so bad. Although they would hesitate to saute something in two tablespoons of butter, they will use four tablespoons of margarine or oil without concern. Another example of this is in the present popular stir-fry method of cooking vegetables in oil. This is a higher fat method of cooking vegetables than plain steaming. People should be aware that it is total fat intake that is important. Equally important is the amount of each form of fat that you use. You can get into trouble by eating too much polyunsaturated fat and very little saturated fat—if you do, your body fat can become abnormally soft. Our bodies need and use both kinds. A recommended ratio is about equal amounts of each.

Recommended Amounts

Nutritionists agree that the amount of fat you should eat daily should be limited. The amount proposed by the Senate Select Committee on Nutrition and Human Needs is 30 percent of your calorie intake. The foods needed for good health supply about 45 grams of fat (see the table on page 178). Since each gram of fat supplies 9 calories, this will supply 405 calories. The total calories from the carbohydrate, protein, and fat in the foods you need is about 1300, which make the proportion from fat about 33 percent. When you add more foods for pleasure and to meet your total energy needs, you should avoid adding them all as fat; carbohydrate foods should be added to keep the proportion of about 30 to 35 percent of your calories from fat, and close to 55 to 60 percent from carbohydrate foods. Usually, getting 10 to 12 percent of calories from protein will meet your protein needs.

Animal and Plant Food Fats

Animal sources of fats include butter, cream, and ice cream—which are all from milk and are not highly processed. Milk fat (cream) is separated from the milk and is then pasteurized or ultrapasteurized. These products contain vitamin A and a small amount of minerals and B-vitamins. Ice cream is lower in fat than light cream and is made in part from whole milk; as a result it is a fair source of calcium. If you are an active person and will use the calories contributed by both the cream and the sugar in ice cream, you can consider it a source of calcium.

Of popular meats in general use, bacon is the highest in fat. It is not highly processed, but it is cured. It contributes protein, niacin, and iron. It also contains nitrite and sodium so it should be used in moderate amounts.

Sardines, sometimes mentioned as a source of calcium, when eaten bones and all are also a good source of protein, potassium, and vitamin A.

Nuts and seeds are also high-fat foods. Instead of using them as snacks, people eating vegetarian meals can use nuts and seeds for amino acids to supplement plant protein. The proteins of nuts lack some of the essential amino acids, but mixtures with foods supplying the missing amino acid can be worked out. Some familiar examples are Chinese vegetable dishes that contain almonds that are eaten with rice, and desserts made of rice, milk, and almonds. Some nuts have a fair protein content in relation to the amount of fat they contain, but for the nonvegetarian the caloric value of nuts is fairly high.

Refined Oils and Fats

Most of the oils on the market today are highly refined to give them non-refrigerated shelf life. The substances that cause natural oils and fats to oxidize at room temperature over a period of time are removed. Some oils and shortenings on the market are as refined a source of fat calories as sugar is a refined source of carbohydrate calories. Some, however, are good sources of vitamin E.

Refined fats and oils go through the following processes. The oils are dissolved out of the original plant or animal material by special solvents, which are then removed from the oil. The crude oil is then treated with a form of soda to remove all free fatty acids, any protein, and other substances. The oil is then bleached by an aluminum compound that picks up the material that gives the oil any color, and also treated with steam to take out any substances that give it undesirable flavors. Following this, it is chilled, and any oil that becomes cloudy is separated from the clear. The clear oil is used as an oil for salad dressings, which then do not become cloudy when refrigerated, as well as for cooking oil. The cloudy oil is used in shortenings and margarines.

Solid Fats from Oils

Shortenings and margarine are made either from a mixture of animal or vegetable fats, and oils, or they may be made only from vegetable oil. Check the label to find out. Oil is hydrogenated to make it solid. Hydrogen is added to the places where there are two bonds in the oil molecule (see Chapter 2, page 28). This changes the oil from a liquid to a solid soft or hard fat, depending on how much it is hydrogenated. The process makes the oil usable in ways other than as just an oil, for example, as margarine or shortening, and also makes it less likely to spoil. It also changes the polyunsaturated fats into saturated ones, which is a disadvantage because some of the essential linoleic acid content of the oil is changed. About 60 percent of all the oil used today in food products is soybean oil. Because it contains a lot of linoleic acid, it spoils very easily; consequently, much of it is hydrogenated. Soybean oil is probably the "hydrogenated vegetable oil" you see listed as an ingredient in convenience foods.

Shortenings

Before the turn of the century, lard and butter were the chief fats used in baking, and in a great deal of other cooking. The first soft shortening came on the market about 1900, and was made of cottonseed oil blended with animal fat. Very soon after this, the process of hydrogenation came into use, and shortenings could be made of only vegetable oils. Cottonseed and corn oils were the first oils used for this. Today, soybean and palm oil have largely replaced cottonseed oil. Until 1961, most shortenings had a low level of polyunsaturated fats (from 5 to 12 percent). Since then, manufacturers have increased the amount, and there are special shortenings on the market that contain 22 to 33 percent polyunsaturated fatty acids.

Margarines

Margarines are made by blending fats or hydrogenated fats and oils with water and milk solids or other milk products. Salt, flavoring, coloring, and vitamins are then added. Unlike shortenings, which have no nutrients other than fat, margarines have some trace of minerals from the added milk products, and they are also fortified with vitamins A and D.

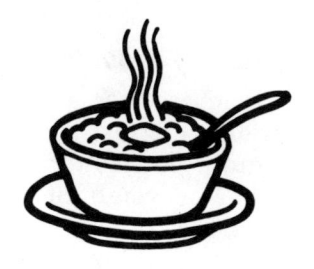

CONSUMER PROTECTION

Dairy Food Fats

There are standards of identity for butter, cream, and ice cream. Ice creams do not have ingredients listed on the carton because they have to be made according to FDA standards or recipes. All commercially available cream is pasteurized or ultra-pasteurized.

Butter

Butter must meet state standards and federal regulations for composition and quality. It is graded by the USDA. Butter is made from pasteurized sweet cream and contains not less than 80 percent milk fat. The cream may be ripened by a lactic acid culture for a short time before churning to develop desirable flavor and aroma. It may also be colored and salted. Butter that has been graded by the USDA has a shield on the package showing the grade. The grade depends on flavor, body, texture, color, and salt content. The grades are AA for the best, then A, B, and C. Butter that has been whipped to incorporate air is usually unsalted.

Cream Products

Heavy cream contains not less than 36 percent butterfat. Light cream contains not less than 18 percent but not more than 30 percent butterfat. Sour cream is pasteurized cream which has been soured by lactic-acid-producing bacteria. It contains not less than 18 percent butterfat. Half-and-half is pasteurized milk and cream which is at least 10.5 percent but not more than 18 percent butterfat. Sour half-and-half is pasteurized half-and-half which has been soured by lactic-acid-producing bacteria. It contains not less than 10.5 percent and not more than 18 percent butterfat.

Dessert Products

Ice cream is made and labeled according to established FDA regulations. It must be made from pasteurized milk products and contain no less than 10 percent butterfat and 20 percent milk solids by weight of the finished ice cream. All ingredients are regulated. If the flavoring, vanilla, for example, is artificial, the ice cream must be labeled "vanilla-flavored" ice cream and not "vanilla" ice cream. French ice cream is made under similar regulations with an increased requirement for egg yolks.

Mellorine is a fabricated frozen dessert also made according to an FDA standard. The basic mix must contain not less than 6 percent fat by weight and 2.7 percent protein from milk. It is sweetened by a nutritive carbohydrate sweetener and fortified with 40 IU of vitamin A for each gram of fat. Flavoring and other ingredients are specified.

Margarine, Mayonnaise, and Salad Dressings

Margarine must meet FDA standards. It must be 80 percent fat, and the fat must be an approved animal fat or vegetable fat or mixture. Water, milk solids, soy protein, and other ingredients that can be used are specified in the regulations. Margarine must have vitamin A added at a level of 15,000 IU per pound, and it *may* have vitamin D added at a level of 1,500 IU per pound. Regular margarine may contain salt, and diet margarine may contain potassium chloride instead of sodium chloride. Margarine may also be colored with carotene. Any preservatives and other allowable ingredients it contains must be listed in order of predominance by weight. Margarines must have nutrition labeling because they are fortified. Margarines may have nutrition information on the fat composition and cholesterol content.

Mayonnaise, salad dressing, and French dressing are high-fat foods that have to be manufactured according to the FDA code of regulations. Mayonnaise does not have to have the ingredients listed on the label, but many companies do so because consumers are not aware that the FDA dictates what must go into a product so that it can be labeled as mayonnaise. The ingredients are similar to those you would find in a recipe: at least 65 percent, by weight of salad oil, not less than 2½ percent vinegar, and egg yolk.

Salad dressings must contain at least 30 percent by weight of vegetable oil, and some egg yolk. Salad dressing contains a cooked or partly cooked starchy paste made of tapioca, wheat, or rye flour, or a combination of any two. The seasonings and other ingredients are specified. French dressing must contain 35 percent by weight of vegetable oil. It also contains vinegar and other allowable ingredients.

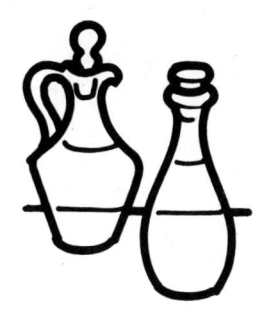

ALCOHOLIC BEVERAGES

		Calories	Alcohol (gm)
Beer	8 oz	110	10
Gin	1½ oz	126	18
Liqueur, cordial	glass	50	7
Vodka	1½ oz	135	19
Whiskey	1½ oz	112	16
Red wine	4 oz	100	12
White wine	4 oz	95	11

NUTRITIVE VALUE OF HIGH-FAT FOODS

			gm	gm	gm	gm	mg	gm	mg
Animal Fats:	Amount	Energy Calories	Carbo-hydrate	Total Fat	Saturated Fatty Acids	Poly-unsaturated Fatty Acids	Cholesterol	Protein	Calcium
Butter	1 tbsp	108	0	12	7.2	.3	33	—	3
Cream, heavy	1 tbsp	80	.4	6	3.5	.1	21	+	10
light	1 tbsp	45	.6	5	2.9	.1	10	+	14
sour	1 tbsp	25	.5	3	1.6	.1	5	+	14
Ice cream, 16% fat	½ c	175	16	12	7.5	.2	44	2	75
soft serve	½ c	185	19	12	7	1	42	3	118
Bacon, fried crisp	2 sl	85	0	8	2.5	1	+	4	2
Sardines	3 oz	175	9	9	3	.5	1	20	372
Vegetable fats:									
Oil, corn	1 tbsp	120	0	14	1.7	8	0	0	0
coconut	1 tbsp	120	0	14	12	.1	0	0	0
peanut	1 tbsp	120	0	14	2.5	4	0	0	0
Margarine, corn oil	1 tbsp	100	0	11	2	4	0	0	0
regular	1 tbsp	100	0	12	3	3	0	0	0
Mayonnaise	1 tbsp	100	.2	11	2	6	7	—	3
Salad dressing	1 tbsp	65	2	6	1.1	3	8	—	2
oil & vinegar type	1 tbsp	85	2	9	1	5	0	—	0
Nuts, almonds, salted	15 nuts	90	30	8	.6	1.1	0	3	35
coconut, shredded	¼ c	181	18	13	12	.1	0	1.2	5
cashews, oil roasted	14 nuts	157	8	13	2.4	1	0	5	11
pecans	10 nuts	69	1.5	7	.4	1	0	1	7
walnuts	5 halves	65	1.6	6	.5	5	0	1.5	10
Seeds, Sesame	⅓ c	290	9	27	3.3	11	0	9	55
Sunflower	⅓ c	271	9.6	23	2.6	9	0	12	58
Coffee whitener, liquid	½ oz	20	0	2	1	+	0	0	1
dry	1 tsp	11	1	1	.6	+	0	+	+

+ Probably present.
— No data.

Phosphorus mg	Sodium mg	Potassium mg	Iron mg	Zinc mg	Vitamin A IU	Vitamin E mg	Thiamin mg	Riboflavin mg	Niacin mg	Vitamin B-6 mg	Folacin mcg	Vitamin D IU
3	123	3	.03	+	459	.15	+	+	+	+	+	+
9	6	11	+	.03	220	.4	+	.02	+	+	1	+
12	6	18	.01	.04	108	.1	+	.02	.01	+	1	+
10	6	17	.01	.03	95	.1	+	.02	.01	+	1	+
57	54	110	.05	.60	448	.1	.02	.14	.57	.02	1	+
101	82	119	.2	.43	395	.1	.04	.27	.1	.06	3	+
36	153	38	.5	.28	0	0	.08	.05	.8	.16	0	—
420	699	502	.3	2.40	190	0	.02	.17	.5	.15	16	420
0	0	0	0	0	0	1.5	0	0	0	0	0	0
0	0	0	0	0	0	—	0	0	0	0	0	0
0	0	0	0	0	0	1.8	0	0	0	0	0	0
0	115	0	0	0	500	1.4	0	0	0	0	0	60
0	115	4	0	0	470	1.4	0	0	0	0	0	60
4	80	0	.1	0	40	2.2	0	0	0	0	0	0
4	110	1	0	0	30	1.1	0	0	0	0	0	0
2	+	2	0	0	0	0	0	0	0	0	0	0
76	30	116	.7	.2	0	2.3	.04	.14	.5	.02	7	0
28	7	116	.7	.9	0	0	.01	.01	.1	.1	8	0
56	2	130	1	.1	28	.8	.12	.07	.5	.06	8	0
—	—	60	.2	—	13	—	.08	.01	.1	—	—	0
28	0	45	.3	.2	3	2.2	.03	.01	.1	.05	5	0
335	20	200	1.2	5	25	—	.09	.07	2.9	—	—	0
—	15	445	3.4	—	23	—	.33	.11	.6	—	—	0
10	12	29	+	+	13	0	0	0	0	0	0	0
8	4	16	+	+	4	0	0	0	0	0	0	0

12.
Convenience Foods

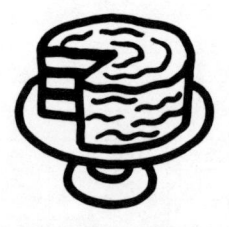

Establishing a supply of food for the city population has been a challenge ever since towns and cities developed. The quality of food and honesty of suppliers have been questioned by city dwellers of every age. Today, we have a remarkable array of foods and food products, the most extensive ever known. At the same time we have extensive suspicion of food products and the producers of them.

The challenge today is for us, the consumers, to make good choices from the proliferation of processed products, especially those containing a great number of additives. The use of a lot of these foods can result in high intake levels that have not been tested for safety in combination.

The thousands of food items on sale in any supermarket are convenient to the extent that you simply have to choose them from the shelves. But by convenience foods we mean foods that have been developed to meet our present day life-style, that take little time and work to prepare. The staples of the present were convenience foods in the past.

Bread, one of the earliest of these, was baked in central bakeries in ancient Rome. Meats were cured and made into dry sausages. The convenient supply of fresh meat such as we have today was only in its beginning when refrigeration machines were invented a hundred years ago. After Pasteur's discoveries of bacteria and of their destruction by heat the canning industry was born. Canned soups and canned tomatoes have been popular convenience foods for over a hundred years.

As trade and the food industry developed many other foods became generally available in the new grocery stores that sold only food and soon replaced the old general store.

CONSUMER PROTECTION

In 1907 the first Pure Food Law was passed to prevent fraud in the manufacture of food products and the sale of foods and products. The law required that all the then familiar products on the market and any new ones coming on the market, had to be wholesome and honest. Over the years Federal regulations that specify the quality and quantity of ingredients allowed in some foods, have been passed. Or standards have been established for some products.

The code of Federal regulations says that all brands of a standardized food must conform to "your image of the food." For example, if a product is labeled "egg noodles," it must contain the same ingredients you would use to make them. A standard of identity specifies the normal composition of the food, the kinds and amounts of ingredients that must go into the product, and certain permissible ingredients that may be added if the manufacturer wishes.

There are 23 classes of foods for which there are established standards; these cover over 200 food products—some of the standards have been covered in the chapters on the specific foods. The 23 classes are as follows:

    Chocolate and cocoa products
    Cereal flours and related products
    Macaroni and noodle products
    Bakery products
    Milk and cream
    Cheese and related cheese foods
    Frozen desserts
    Food flavoring
    Dressings for food
    Nutritive sweeteners
    Canned fruit and fruit juices
    Fruit pies
    Fruit butters, preserves and related products
    Table syrup
    Nonalcoholic beverages

Canned shellfish and fish
Eggs and egg products
Margarines
Nut products
Frozen vegetables
Canned vegetables
Tomato products
Foods for special dietary uses

Food Laws: A Safe Food Supply

In addition to the establishment of standards there have been laws enacted to guarantee the safety of our food supply.

In 1938 the Pure Food and Cosmetic Act required "pure wholesome food," honest labeling, and packaging. In 1954 the Pesticide Amendment established the amount of residues of pesticides that are allowed to remain on fresh agricultural commodities shipped interstate. It must not be above a level proven to be safe by both scientific evaluations and tests on animals.

In 1958 the Food Additives Amendment was passed, requiring proof of safety before a substance may be added to a food. It also allows food companies to modify the food supply by permitting the use of substances which are safe at the levels of intended use. One of the most important parts of this amendment is the much-discussed Delaney clause:

> An additive is prohibited if it causes cancer to develop in any experimental animal when fed to the animal in any amount whatsoever.

In 1960, substances used for color in foods were regulated by another amendment to the 1938 law. Regulations regarding the possibility that the color could cause cancer are the same as those in the Food Additive Amendment.

REGULATED ADDITIVES

The substances that may be added to foods are divided into two groups. One group consists of the newly developed additives (regulated); the other of substances which have been in use for a long time; they are called the Generally Recognized as Safe List (GRAS).

The newly developed additives must be tested for safety before they can be used. The testing requires that the substance be fed to at least two species of animals through at least two generations. The amount allowed for humans is usually 1/100 of the maxiumum amount safe for the animals. In addition to the safety level, the food company must show that the additive will accomplish the purpose for which it is added to the food, and that the amount they propose to use is no more than is needed for that purpose. It is important to note, however, that additives are not tested in combination with one another.

Over the years that people have been cooking and preserving foods, many substances have been used. Sugar is one of the most common preservatives, salt and saltpeter have been used in curing meat for centuries. These and others such as pepper, spices, and even vegetables when used for flavoring, and all substances that were generally recognized as safe, made up the first GRAS list. Since the list was first drawn up, some of the items on it have been tested and banned from use, and new ones have been added. The list now consists of 675 items.

Purposes of Additives

An incidental additive is one that is allowed in foods in the least possible amount and comes from the production and handling of foods or food components. Pesticide residues and detergent residues from washing processing equipment are examples.

An intentional additive is allowed to be added to a food only if it has a purpose—such as improving the nutritional quality, keeping quality, or stability, making the food attractive; aid in processing; or providing a component for a special diet. It cannot be used if it is hazardous to health, lowers nutritive value, disguises faulty processing or poor quality food, or deceives the consumer. It cannot be used if the same effect can be obtained by other, nonadditive processes.

Intentional additives must not be added in quantities more than needed to do the job. They must conform to an approved standard for purity and must be tested for safety. Approval for use of an additive is limited to specific foods for specific purposes. Some additives can be used only for foods used by special groups.

Flavor

Most intentional additives (a large part of the GRAS list) are those added for flavor. Many of these substances are not generally thought of as additives, such as spices, herbs, and flavorings used in foods; and many are the ground spices and oils extracted from the natural sources. Some are synthetic. Some, such as monosodium glutamate, are flavor enhancers.

Preventing Spoilage

Foods lose quality or become unsafe to eat because of changes within the foods themselves or because bacteria or molds develop. Additives called antioxidants prevent changes within the food itself. Antioxidants, such as butylated-hydroxy anisole (BHA), prevent fats from becoming rancid, and are added to oils, salad dressings, fried foods, potato chips, cake mixes (because they contain shortening), margarines, baked goods, and most convenience products that contain fats.

Other antioxidants are added to keep peeled and cut fruits from turning brown. The most used additive for this purpose is ascorbic acid (vitamin C). Sulphur dioxide is used to prevent darkening of dried fruits. Additives that prevent molds from growing are used in bread and bakery products, cheese products, syrups, candy, jams, and jellies. Sugar is the oldest such additive. Still other additives such as salt and sodium nitrite prevent harmful bacteria from developing in salted and cured meats. Sodium benzoate is used for the same purpose in margarine, fruit juices, and pickled vegetables.

Nutritive Value

Following the assurance that our foods are safe to eat, our next prime concern is their nutritive value: Mineral and vitamin additives are added to foods under the regulations for enrichment. The first regulation was the enrichment of bread in 1941. It was extended in 1961 and revised in 1968 and 1973. It endorses:

- Enrichment of flour, bread, degerminated cornmeal, corn grits, wholegrain cornmeal, white rice and certain other cereal products with thiamin, riboflavin, niacin, and iron.
- Fortification of milk, fluid skim milk, and nonfat dry milk with vitamin D.
- Fortification of margarine, fluid skim milk, and nonfat dry milk with vitamin A.

- Addition of potassium iodide to table salt.
- Standardized addition of fluoride to water in areas where water supply has low fluoride content because the protective action of fluoride against dental caries is recognized.

Nutrients can be added to other foods without rigid regulations; for example, the addition of vitamin C to fruit juices and artificially colored and flavored fruit drinks and the addition of protein and many vitamins and minerals to cereals and quick breakfast pastries.

Texture and Consistency

The additives that are used to give or maintain texture can be divided, according to function, into three groups—emulsifiers, stabilizers, and thickeners. Some additives can perform all three functions. Emulsifiers keep ingredients from separating. They are used by the baking industry to make batters and doughs easier to handle and to produce volume and fine grain. They are used in some shortenings and cake mixes so cakes with a higher ratio of sugar to flour can be made. Emulsifiers keep chocolate candy from changing color if it becomes warm, and they act as flavor carriers in candies. They are also used to keep ice cream and other frozen desserts smooth and creamy because they help mixtures of fats and other liquids to mix and stay mixed.

Stabilizers also keep ingredients from separating. They keep solids from separating from liquids and are used in chocolate milk. They make ice cream smoother, with finer ice crystals. Stabilizers also prevent flavors from being lost from cake and pudding mixes. Thickeners are used to give body or greater consistency. They include starches, pectins, cellulose products, vegetable gums, agar, alginates, and carrageenans.

Chemical Reactions

Called by their common names, many substances in this group of additives are familiar. Food acids such as lemon juice (citric acid) and vinegar (acetic acid) are used to provide flavor and texture in some products. Fruit acids are used in jams and jellies, and vinegar is used in pickles and salad dressings; these may also be used in other products where a tart flavor is desired. Cream is "soured" by lactic acid, and sometimes butter is made from cream slightly soured in this way for better flavor. Phosphoric acid is used in some soft drinks.

Alkaline substances are used as leavening agents. Baking soda is sodium bicarbonate, and baking powders are blends of soda with salts which have names like potassium acid tartrate and sodium aluminum phosphate. Special baking powder combinations have been developed for cake, pancake, muffin, and biscuit mixes. One alkaline substance, sodium hydroxide, is used for the glaze on pretzels.

Color

Many foods have bright and pleasing colors in nature, and food colors used to be derived from plant sources. As the number of convenience products increased, the supply of natural coloring became insufficient, so synthetics were developed. About 90 percent of all colors now in use are synthetic. They are used for ice cream, soft drinks, gelatin desserts, meat casings, pudding mixes, and some bakery products. Margarines and dairy products are usually colored by the natural color carotene.

Improvers (flour and bread)

Freshly milled flour does not produce as fine baked products as flour that has been allowed to "age." Aged flour is whiter in color. Because aging is a slow process when allowed to proceed at a natural rate and during aging flour can deteriorate and become infested by insects, today millers use maturing and bleaching agents to produce flour of good color and good baking qualities almost immediately after milling. Bread improvers and yeast foods that bakers are allowed to use produce breads of uniform quality.

Removing Trace Minerals

Additives called sequestrants seek out and combine with substances that might affect the keeping qualities of a product. They are used mostly to combine with copper and other trace minerals in fats. These nutrients act as catalysts in causing fats to go rancid. Sequestrants are also used by soft-drink manufacturers to make the water clear.

Additives to Keep Foods Moist

Humectants are added, for example, to brown sugar and dried coconut to keep them moist.

Additives to Keep Salt Free Flowing

Anticaking agents are added to salt, flavored salts, powdered sugar, and malted milk powder to keep these products dry.

Additives to Firm Up Foods

Firming agents are used to improve the texture of processed fruits and vegetables. Canned tomatoes, for example, which years ago were very soft, now hold their shape. Canned peas, potatoes, and apples are also treated with these agents.

Additives to Make Liquids Clear

These are similar in action to sequestrants and are used to remove trace minerals that would cause liquids to become cloudy.

Others

Additives are used to prevent foaming during the process of canning or bottling some juices such as orange juice and pineapple juice. Foaming agents make pressure-packed whipped toppings squirt out of their containers. Non-nutritive sweeteners give a chemical sweetness to foods for people who do not want to consume the 13 calories in a teaspoon of sugar.

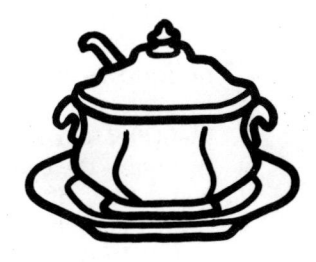

WEIGHING NUTRITION AGAINST CONVENIENCE

Through the development of intentional additives food technologists employed by food companies have been able to produce synthetic counterparts of substances in foods to modify or replace naturally occurring ingredients. This has provided us with a vast selection of foods with long shelf life and with products that could not otherwise exist. Intentional additives are used mostly in packaged products that keep at ordinary temperatures, although an increasing number of frozen entrees and vegetables with sauces require additives to maintain texture and quality. These practices may not all be to our nutritional advantage.

Self-rising flour (flour combined with baking powder) was one of the first old-style convenience foods to be changed to a new-style convenience product. Baking-powder biscuit mix was created by adding shortening to the flour mixture. In its early days it had a limited shelf life because the fine particles of shortening became rancid. From this beginning, a whole group of mixes containing fats or fat substances, with equal likelihood of going rancid, was developed. Cake mixes and brown-and-serve products would have short shelf life without the additives in them.

Checking Ingredients

As more and more products in which ingredients are already combined were developed, more and more additives were used to prevent decline in quality. Consumers enjoyed the convenience of these quick and easy-to-make foods but began raising questions about the "chemicals" they heard were being added to them. This resulted in 1968 in the passage of The Fair Packaging and Labeling Law, with its ingredient-listing regulations. The following information must be on the label:

1. Identification of the product by its usual name.
2. Weight of the contents and the number of servings.
3. Name and address of the manufacturer.
4. Ingredients in the product listed in descending order by weight (if it is a food without a Federal standard).

As was mentioned in the chapter on cereals, the listing by weight can give a different impression of the contents of major ingredients when you are used to measuring by volume when you cook. In manufacturing the ingredients are measured by weight as it is more accurate.

Additives are used in such small amounts, and the amounts allowed are so regulated, that the fact that they are listed is as important as the order. However, if you are on a low-salt diet you should look at how many ingredients contain sodium.

Since January 1978, the reason an additive is in a product must also be given. This does not change the fact, however, that some of the additives are foreign substances.

Making a Choice

The consumption of additives is the trade-off you make for your time and labor in food preparation. You have the ultimate power of choice over these products. Many products have come on the market and disappeared because they did not catch on. The one message the manufacturer will always hear is that a product did not sell. If you feel strongly against the use of additives, there are still many foods available in which few or none are used. Even if you are not particularly concerned and feel that the FDA is a trustworthy watchdog, it is probably a good idea not to rely too heavily on foods containing many such substances, and to balance your food intake with fresh, home-cooked foods.

It's important to know how a convenience food compares in nutritive value with the homemade product made from fresh ingredients. For example, pizza made from a home recipe of enriched flour and yeast contains a certain amount of the B-vitamins. The tomato paste contains vitamin C and the cheese many nutrients, as does the meat or fish if it is added. When baked at the high temperature required, there are vitamin losses; but there are no further losses if you eat it right away. Frozen pizza, however, loses thiamin and ascorbic acid in freezer storage. Since you have to reheat it, there is further loss of vitamins. While freshly baked pizza has a certain vitamin C value, the reheated baked product probably has very little.

If you compare the ingredient listing on a convenience product and the recipe in a good cookbook, you will be able to tell how they match up to each other. If they are quite similar, the nutritive value will also be similar.

Fresh, Canned, and Dehydrated Soups

In comparing fresh and canned soups, you may find that the ingredient lists are fairly similar. The nutritive values are also fairly similar. However, with dehydrated soup products, which may be pleasing appetizers, you will find varying caloric and nutrient values. You must look at the ingredients in them before assuming them to be equal to homemade conventional foods; they are not equal.

CREAM OF TOMATO SOUP

	Fresh (Homemade)	Canned
Ingredients	1 cup chopped fresh tomatoes ¼ cup chopped celery 2 tbsp chopped onion 1 tsp sugar 1 tsp salt ⅛ tsp pepper 2 tbsp butter 2 tbsp flour	Tomatoes Vitamin C Citric acid Sugar Salt Natural spice oils Vegetable oil Enriched wheat flour
Preparation	Tomatoes, celery, and onion are seasoned with sugar, salt, and pepper, cooked to a puree, then thickened with flour.	Tomatoes are cooked to a puree then cooked with other ingredients in the can.
Time involved	Puree takes about 30 minutes to cook.	It takes about 30 seconds to open can.
Serving instructions	Add 2 cups milk or milk and cream and heat.	Add 1 can milk and heat.

Dehydrated

Dehydrated tomato powder
Dehydrated onion
Garlic powder
Sugar
Salt
Hydrogenated vegetable oil
Food starch, modified
Soy flour
Cornstarch
Natural flavor
Artificial flavors
Lactose
Sodium caseinate
Monosodium glutamate
Dipotassium phosphate
Mono- and di-glycerides
Artificial color
Chicken fat
Freeze-dried chicken meat
Thiamin hydrochloride (B_1)
Sodium silico aluminate
Disodium inosinate
Disodium guanylate
Tricalcium phosphate
Lecithin
Tumeric
Corn-syrup solids
Polysorbate
Spices

Make soup with water.

Heat and serve according to package directions.

Evaluating Frozen Meals

Among the most popular of all convenience foods are frozen entrees, frozen entrees with potatoes or pasta, and frozen dinners. In reheating these products nutrients sensitive to heat, such as vitamin C and thiamin, can be lost. There is some loss of magnesium when the vegetable of a frozen dinner is blanched before processing, and there is gradual loss of vitamin B_6 in the meat during freezer storage.

Frozen Heat-and-Serve Dinner Guidelines

There are recently established "nutritional quality guidelines" for "heat-and-serve" dinners. These guidelines may be used by a manufacturer on a voluntary basis. The way you can tell is by looking for the following statement on the label: "This product provides nutrients in amounts appropriate for this class of food as determined by the U.S. Government." To be labeled as a frozen heat-and-serve dinner, the product must contain "three components, one of which is a significant source of protein." The three components must consist of one or more of the following: meat, poultry, fish, cheese, eggs, vegetables, fruit, potatoes, rice, or other cereal-based products. It may also contain soup, rolls, dessert, or beverage. The dinner may be named by the protein source, such as "frozen chicken dinner"; and the other components may be given in descending order by weight.

To meet the nutritional guidelines, frozen dinners must consist of three components: (1) a source of protein from meat, poultry, fish, cheese, or eggs that supplies 70 percent of the total protein of the dinner; (2) one or more vegetables or vegetable mixtures other than potatoes, rice, or a cereal-based product; (3) potatoes, rice, or a cereal-based product (other than bread or rolls), or another vegetable or combination of vegetables. The three components have to provide certain nutrients at levels set by the FDA. The dinner will be prepared from conventional foods and also contain folic acid, magnesium, iodine, calcium, and zinc. The nutrients must come from the three main foods, although soup, rolls, dessert, and beverage may be included.

Frozen and Fresh Vegetables

Some vegetables and cereals are made to cook quickly by the

addition of alkaline salts to soften the fiber. This technique can lower the vitamin content.

The ingredients of a fresh vegetable dish compared with those in a similar frozen dish are listed below.

Sweet and Sour Vegetables

Carrots
Green pepper
Tomatoes
Green beans
Pineapple cubes

Sauce
  Syrup from canned pineapple
  Molasses
  Brown sugar

  Corn starch
  Soy sauce
  Chicken-flavored bouillon
    cubes
  Vinegar

Frozen Hawaiian Vegetables

Carrots
Celery
Pineapple
White onions
Pea pods

Sauce
  Water
  Pineapple juice
  Sugar
  Peanut oil
  Cornstarch, modified
  Soy sauce
  Chicken-flavored bouillon
  Sherry concentrate
  Salt
  Garlic powder

The recipe using fresh food takes considerable time to prepare. The vegetables take time to cook and the sauce has to be made separately. The frozen product compares favorably, and if it has been carefully handled as a perishable but frozen food, it should have an equally favorable nutritive value. The preservation of this product is by freezing alone, although the acidity and vitamin C in the pineapple juice helps prevent loss of flavors and vitamins.

Baked Goods

As shown below, a homemade poundcake and one made from a cake mix differ in the kind of shortening and the number of eggs. This makes a difference in vitamin A and iron values. The mix is not a true poundcake; the emulsified shortening gives volume without the half-pound of eggs and permits a higher sugar level.

Classic Poundcake Recipe

½ pound sugar (1 cup)
½ pound butter (1 cup)
½ pound flour (2 cups)
½ pound eggs (6 eggs)
1 teaspoon vanilla
½ teaspoon baking powder
   (optional in some recipes)

Poundcake Mix

Sugar
Emulsified shortening
Enriched flour, corn flour
Salt
Nonfat milk solids
Artificial flavor
Baking powder

Make with 2 eggs and ¾ cup whole milk.

Though today we don't usually think of cake as a source of nutrients but more a food for pleasure, in times when there was less food available, all food eaten contributed to the supply of nutrients. We must retain this concept. We cannot eat low-nutrient foods with about the same calories and keep healthy.

Some popular cakes could not exist without the use of additives. The party cake below is an available product. The nutritive value is questionable. From such a product, it is a small step to fabricated foods.

Chocolate Cake (Recipe)

(Made with butter, milk, and 2 eggs)

Sugar
Enriched bleached flour
Butter or margarine

Dutch-type cocoa
Baking powder
Salt

Milk

Vanilla extract

Party Cake (Ingredients)

Made with ½ cup butter, margarine, or oil, water, and 2 eggs)

Sugar
Enriched bleached flour
Shortening with mono- and di-glycerides, BHA, BHT, citric acid
Cocoa processed with alkali
Leavening
Salt
Propylene glycol mono esters (for moistness)
Soy flour
Soy protein concentrate
Modified tapioca starch
Cellulose
Tragacanth gums
Artificial flavor

Coconut Macaroon (Filling)
Sugar
Flour
Coconut
Corn starch
(A soft macaroon would contain the above ingredients, but would probably not bake as the filling in the mix does.)

Glaze
Butter or margarine
Confectioners' sugar
Vanilla extract
Milk or water

Filling (Made with water)
Sugar
Enriched bleached flour
Coconut
Shortening (additives as above)
Corn sugar
Leavening
Soy flour
Salt
Propylene glycol monoesters
Natural and artificial flavoring

Glaze (Made with water)
Sugar
Vegetable shortening
Wheat starch
Modified tapioca starch
Salt
Mono- and di-glycerides
Poly sorbate 80
Artificial color
Artificial flavor

USING SNACK FOODS AND FABRICATED FOODS

Snack foods belong to a group of new convenience foods that are designed with no nutritional concept in mind. Sales were nearly a billion dollars in 1976. Snack foods, or so-called fun foods, are convenient for nibbling as one sits watching television or conversing in social groups. They are also convenient sources of calories and, often, salt.

A good common-sense rule to follow is to eat only the foods that are the backbone of good nutrition for a day or two following a day of eating for sociability. In this way, you will use the calories your efficient physiological system stored up, and you will not accumulate fat reserves. You cannot interfere with the body mechanisms that store calories without perhaps causing injury to your health. But you can always use up the calories by allowing your body's automatic mechanism to call on fat reserves for energy whenever you spend more energy.

Fabricated foods are products that have been developed as replacements for traditional foods. The groups listed below belong to this class.

Coffee Whiteners and Imitation Milk

Products to be added to coffee in place of cream or milk come in both liquid and dry form. The liquids keep longer than fresh cream under refrigeration; they are used a great deal in food service operations, especially in meals on airplanes. They can be frozen and kept for long periods and when thawed will keep several weeks in the refrigerator. Dry coffee whiteners can be kept at room temperature (on kitchen shelves or in office desk drawers) for quite a long time without changing. These products are made of a non-dairy fat, usually coconut oil; a protein substance, either sodium caseinate from milk or a soy protein; a sweetener, such as corn syrup; emulsifiers; buffers; and stabilizers. They have a high sodium content. They are designed as a flavorful replacement for cream in coffee but not for food value. People often use them believing that the vegetable oil, as listed, will provide polyunsaturated fat, but coconut oil actually provides saturated fat. People are mistaken in thinking these products are better than cream because they are made of vegetable fat.

Imitation milk products are made of ingredients similar to those in coffee whiteners. They have to be called "imitation" because they do not have the nutritive value of milk.

Instant Liquid Meals

There is a varied selection of products designed to take the place of a meal, usually on the basis of lowered calories. These "meals" may have a poor balance of trace minerals and vitamins. They certainly lack fiber. The ingredients and nutritive value vary with the brand.

Whipped Toppings

Whipped toppings are similar to coffee whiteners. They may have a base of nonfat dry milk with added vegetable oil. They come dry, in pressurized cans, or already whipped and frozen. Ingredients might be hydrogenated coconut and palm kernel oil, sugar, corn syrup, dextrose, sodium caseinate, polysorbate 60, natural and artificial colors, sorbutan monostearate, xanathan gum, guar gum, and artificial color.

Fruit Drinks

Many fruit drinks are not the nutrient equivalents of fresh fruits except in their added vitamin C or ascorbic acid.

Imitation Bacon Bits

The word "imitation" means that fabricated bacon bits do not have the nutritive value of pork bacon bits. They are made of defatted soy flour, vegetable shortening containing the partly hydrogenated oils of soy and cotton seed, salt, natural and artificial flavor, water, sugar, and artificial color.

Meat Analogs

Some products made from textured soy protein are colored and treated to resemble meats. Major minerals and vitamins are sometimes added in the proportions present in real meat. Soy concentrate sticks, which resemble frankfurters, have the highest consumer acceptance in this group of products.

Breakfast Cereals and Pastries

Some breakfast cereals are so processed as to qualify more as fabricated foods than as cereals. They are usually made of flour and starch rather than whole grain, and they sometimes contain marshmallow-like candy bits. The ingredient listing may include oat flour, sugar, corn syrup, corn starch, dextrose, wheat starch, salt, gelatin, calcium carbonate, sodium phosphate, and natural and artificial colors as well as a list of the added vitamins or their compounds—sodium ascorbate, niacin, vitamin A palmitate, pyridoxine hydrochloride, riboflavin, thiamin, mononitrate, cyancobalamin, vitamin D_2. (For information on how to judge a breakfast cereal, see Chapter 10.)

Breakfast pastries are similar fabricated foods.

13.

How To Choose a Nutritionally Balanced Diet

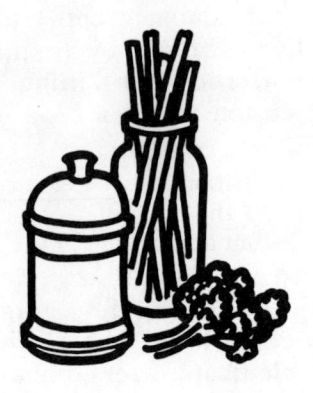

A balanced diet supplies all the nutrients essential to your health from a variety of foods in realistic amounts. You must eat some foods daily and some at least each week. With our abundant and varied food supply, you should not need highly fortified foods if you learn which traditional foods will protect your health. Good nutrition is a life-long process. If you do not follow good food rules when you are young, it is difficult to make it up. You will be more likely to have greater vigor and better health as you advance in years if you follow good rules throughout your life.

In the 1940s the specific foods that supplied the then-known nutrients were called "protective foods," or the "basic seven." The naturally occurring foods were divided into seven groups, each of which contributed a high percentage of the known nutrients: the milk group; the protein (animal and vegetable) group; fruits and vegetables high in vitamin A; fruits and vegetables high in vitamin C; potatoes and other vegetables and fruits; foods from grains; and the food fats.

Even though our knowledge of known nutrients and number of new essential nutrients increased, the number of basic groups used as a guide to good nutrition was decreased from seven to four. The basic four groups are: the milk group; the protein group; the fruits and vegetables (with emphasis on those high in vitamins A and C); and the cereal group. The concept of the basic four is too simple for several reasons.

- It ignores fats as a group. It is estimated that 40 percent of the calories in our diets comes from fats, and nutrition authorities recommend that no more than 30 to 35 percent come from fats. This level still permits one-third of our daily calorie intake to come from foods not recognized as a basic group.

- Today there are many "convenience" products on the market that are not equivalents of traditional foods from the standpoint of nutritional values. For example, tomato soup made from a basic recipe includes milk and tomatoes. If it is not heated too long it will have the nutritional value of the two foods, including the vitamin C. On the other hand, tomato soup made from a dehydrated product and water, which may be a pleasing hot appetizer, does not make the major nutritional contribution of the soup from fresh ingredients.

- There has been a change in the methods by which food preparation is taught in schools. In many cases, the school period has been shortened so that the teacher resorts to using "convenience" products. Students may not be taught the nutritional value of fresh foods. Surveys show that many teenage students shop for household foods, if their mothers work, and base their choices on products they like rather than the nutritional needs of family members.

The backbone of good nutrition is made up of traditional foods that can be eaten in reasonable servings and that supply the essential nutrients in fairly high amounts. (See table, page 206.) The nutrients contributed by each of the foods add up to approximately what we need daily. You don't have to calculate your nutrient intake each day from food tables. Rather the food tables are intended to present as complete a profile of the foods as possible, so that you can make comparisons among them. A wide selection of foods is desirable for variety, but in making the selection, compare them so that you get a similar variety of the almost 50 nutrients you need. The foods you choose daily may meet your needs approximately but over the week they should meet your full requirements.

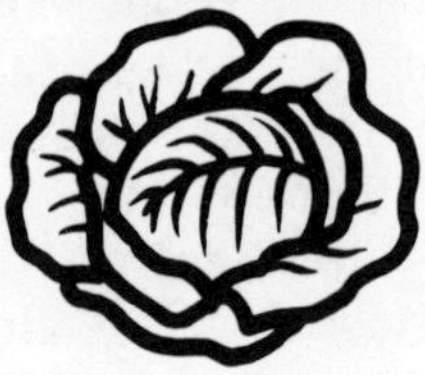

CHOOSE FOODS FOR NUTRIENTS

Calories, those numbers most of us are so conscious of, are really the last factor to consider when choosing foods for their contribution to your health. Calories are important, but just as a measure of energy. Only after you have added up the calories supplied by the foods that meet all your needs for all the nutrients should you consider additional foods to meet your energy or calorie requirement.

Calcium is the first nutrient to consider. There are fewer foods that contain calcium than there are food sources of any other nutrient, so it is the hardest to obtain unless you use the best sources, milk or cheese. Certain fruits, vegetables, and nuts supply amounts of calcium that also count. On a day-to-day basis, milk is the best and most versatile high-calcium food. Milk also supplies protein, riboflavin, vitamin A, vitamin D, vitamin B_{12}, thiamin, phosphorus, and other minerals and vitamins. In the table on page 206, there is some nutrient contribution from milk in every space. Although the table contains only 25 nutrients, it is likely that as a traditional food supporting animal growth it can supply some of all the essential nutrients. An adult needs two glasses of milk each day, or a glass of milk and 1 ounce of cheese, or two ounces of cheese. The major contributions of two glasses of milk are shown below.

Milk	Calcium	Phosphorus	Protein	Vitamin A	Vitamin B_{12}	Riboflavin
	gm.	gm.	gm.	I.U.	mcg.	mg.
16 ounces (2 glasses)	582	456	16	614	1.8	.80

Protein, iron, zinc and vitamin B_{12} are the next nutrients to consider. Although milk and cheese make quite a contribution to our protein need, they are low in iron and zinc. No one food in nature supplies all needed nutrients. The favorite high-protein foods for people other than vegetarians are meat, poultry, and fish. These also contribute iron and zinc. Eggs are the protein food with the best assortment of amino acids of all foods; they are a rich source of iron, vitamin A, the B vitamins and contribute many minerals. The high-protein vegetable foods are lower in protein, high in iron, and contain no fat, an advantage over meat. Some of the nutrients in these foods are listed in the table below.

	Calcium	Phosphorus	Protein	Vitamin A	Vitamin B_{12}	Riboflavin	Iron	Zinc
COMBINATION I	gm.	gm.	gm.	I.U.	mcg.	mg.	mg.	mg.
Milk (16 oz.)	582	456	16	614	1.8	.80	0.2	1.8
Meat (3½ oz.)	10	191	30	50	2.0	.40	4.0	6.0
	592		46		3.8		4.2	7.8
COMBINATION II								
Milk (16 oz.)	582	456	16	614	1.8	.80	0.2	1.8
2 Eggs	56	180	12	520	1.2	.30	2.0	1.4
Legumes (¾ cup)	130	219	12	113	0.	.10	3.8	2.3
	768	855	40		3.0		6.0	5.5

Each of the combinations above includes the milk you need and will meet both your calcium and protein needs almost completely, but not your other nutrient needs. If you eat meat or eggs with beans, your vitamin B_{12} needs are also met. If you eat only beans you will require more milk or cheese for vitamin B_{12}. If you eat only meat, you will require more calcium. When you look at the complete table you will note that these foods contribute practically no vitamin C.

202. *The No-Nonsense Guide to Food and Nutrition*

Vitamin C, potassium, and other macro- and trace minerals are the next nutrients needed toward completion of nutrient needs. We need one food that is an excellent source, or two that are good sources of vitamin C each day. They can be either fruits or vegetables. Naturally occurring foods always contribute potassium, some iron and calcium, many trace elements and some B-vitamins. In choosing a source of vitamin C it isn't a good idea to select a synthetic food that contains only vitamin C. For comparison, look at the nutrient profile of orange juice in the table on page 154. And if you eat an orange, you will also get fiber.

Vitamin A, folacin and other B-vitamins, and minerals are present in the foods discussed above, but not in sufficient amounts to meet your RDA. Milk and egg yolk contribute vitamin A, but we need a fruit or vegetable that is an excellent source of vitamin A along with additional minerals, folacin, and fiber. Look at the nutrient profile of broccoli in the table on page 156 and note (below) its contribution of vitamin C, potassium, and folacin as well as the vitamin A. To ensure an intake of more of the trace minerals, B-vitamins and fiber, both the basic four and basic seven food rules add two more servings of fruits or vegetables. If you have no digestive problems, eating some raw guarantees against cooking losses. The following table includes apple and zucchini, the former appetizing raw or cooked, the latter better cooked. Neither are particularly high in any one nutrient. For the nutritive values of other fruits and vegetables see the tables in Chapter 9.

In looking at the totals, the amount of vitamin C is well

		Vitamin A	Vitamin C	Potassium	Magnesium	Iron	Zinc	Folacin	Thiamin
		I.U.	mg.	mg.	mg.	mg.	mg.	mcg.	mg.
Milk	16 oz.	614	0	740	66	.2	1.8	24	.2
Meat	3½ oz.	50	0	261	21	4.0	6.0	4	.1
Orange Juice	¾ c.	370	83	381	19	.4	.04	102	.17
Broccoli	⅔ c.	2500	90	267	24	.8	.2	56	.09
Apple	1	90	4	100	8	.3	.05	8	.03
Zucchini	1 cup	780	20	282	32	.8	.8	22	.11
TOTALS		4404	197	2031	170	6.5	8.89	216	.79

above the recommended daily allowance for everyone, the vitamin A is well above the RDA for women and children, and the zinc is near the requirements. But there is only half the iron needed and the B-vitamins other than B_{12} do not meet requirements.

The foods from grains complete our nutrient needs, except for essential fatty acids, Vitamin E, iodine, and fluorine. Food rules suggest four servings of whole grain or enriched cereals daily, which, with the above foods more than meet protein needs. However, we suggest a fifth serving of the grain foods for their B-vitamin and mineral contributions and because they are a non-fat source of additional calories. Although Federal regulations mandate that three B-vitamins and iron be added to refined cereals, breads, and pasta, whole grains have other nutrients that are removed in refining. Zinc is one of those removed which is sometimes added to fortified cereals. Zinc is a logical addition, but adding nutrients such as vitamins D and A not present in the original grains is not. The following table shows the contribution of the grain foods to the foods already discussed.

	Thiamin	Riboflavin	Niacin	Vitamin B_6	Folacin	Pantothenic Acid	Iron	Zinc
	mg.	mg.	mg.	mg.	mcg.	mg.	mg.	mg.
Milk (16 oz.)	.2	.8	.4	.2	24	1.6	.2	1.8
Meat (3½ oz.)	.1	.4	4.5	.4	4	.5	4.0	6.0
Fruits, 4 servings vegetables	.4	.4	3.2	.4	188	1.8	2.3	1.09
Hot cereal 1 cup	.15	.05	1.5	.1	118	.2	1.2	1.2
Bread 3 slices	.27	.09	2.4	.1	48	.5	2.4	1.5
Pasta 1 cup	.23	.13	1.8	.1	13	.3	1.4	.7
TOTAL	1.35	1.87	13.8	1.3	395	4.9	11.5	12.29
Potato, baked 1	.15	.06	2.5	.35	26	.6	1.0	.5

Grain foods are easy to include by eating a serving of cereal and a slice of toast for breakfast, a sandwich or pasta for lunch, and pasta or rice for dinner. Because potatoes are a more traditional food for many people, we have shown some of their nutrient values below the table.

Our needs for the essential fatty acids are met by adding to the above essential foods a tablespoon of corn oil or of margarine made with liquid corn oil, along with the contributions of the other foods. We get iodine from iodized salt, if not from seafood or fish, and fluorine in our water supply.

When you compare the totals of the nutrients in the essential foods with the RDA's, you will see they are met except for zinc and vitamin E for the man and woman, except also iron for the woman of child-bearing age. But remember the RDA's have a margin of safety above actual need. However, including liver in your diet, possibly once a week, using some wheat germ, especially if you use enriched processed cereals, and the use of leafy greens in salads with an oil dressing will assure a weekly average meeting your needs.

In addition to the nutrients in the table on page 96, you can turn to the list of dietary essentials tabulated on page 16, Chapter 1 and observe that there are other vitamins and trace minerals included. For vitamin K, biotin, and choline, intestinal synthesis supplies body need as well as traditional foods. For trace minerals, cobalt is covered by adequate vitamin B_{12}, and sulphur by adequate protein. For chromium, manganese, selenium, tin, vanadium, silicon, molybdenum, and nickel we lack knowledge of their quantitative requirement and sources in food. Probably these trace minerals are ensured by the use of naturally occurring protective foods.

We mentioned earlier that there are dangers of overconsumption of food as well as underconsumption in America today. These include excess calories and too much saturated fat and animal protein, cholesterol, sucrose (table sugar), and sodium.

In the basic diet pattern suggested here there are no excesses of saturated fat or animal protein. Lean meat in moderate quantity alternates with poultry, fish, and high-protein vegetable foods. Even an occasional egg used as a protein alternate contains only 252 mg of cholesterol, which is below 300 mg daily, as suggested by the U.S. Dietary Goals of the Select Subcommittee on Nutrition of the U.S. Senate. Non-fat milk can be substituted for whole milk. There is no sucrose in the basic foods and no excess of sodium. Use of table salt (sodium chloride) with added iodine is desirable in moderation, especially if little seafood or fish is used. Sodium is an essential mineral, although too much is undesirable. You are the one who must monitor total calories to avoid overweight. If you already have a health problem, special dietary precautions may be prescribed by your physician, but that is beyond the scope of this book.

NUTRITION AND CALORIES (ENERGY)

The foods that make up the backbone of good nutrition also supply energy—about 1300 calories. The foods you choose as alternatives to those listed should be chosen for similar nutrient contribution. You cannot trade off these foods with any others on the basis of calories alone and be well nourished. The first 1300 calories' worth of foods you eat each day should come from these high-nutrient foods or other foods that supply many nutrients in proportion to the energy they yield.

You have a basic energy requirement of about 1300 calories for the work of your heart, lungs, and other vital life processes. The need is less for small women and men and more for large women and men. The number of additional calories you need a day is the result of your own decisions and activities. If you walk to the next bus stop before boarding you use more body energy. If you walk up a flight of stairs it is not only good for your heart and leg muscles but uses energy. The only way to recognize your energy needs is to watch your weight. Watching your weight does not mean running to the scales every morning, but taking a good look at yourself once every three to four months. If you notice a bulge here and there, it is time to eat fewer low-nutrient extras and lose the bulges. On the other hand, if you notice your waistband is loose or you look thin, it is time to eat more food.

The Backbone of Good Nutrition for an adult is the following foods in these amounts:
  2 cups of milk or 2 ounces of cheese
  1 serving of meat (3½ ounces) or equivalent)
  1 high vitamin A fruit or vegetable
  1 high vitamin C fruit or vegetable
  2 other vegetables or fruits
  1 serving of potato
  4 servings of whole grain or enriched cereal or bread
  1 tablespoon corn oil or corn oil margarine

These foods can be prepared in any ethnic tradition.

THE BACKBONE OF GOOD NUTRITION

	Amount	Calcium (mg)	Phosphorus (mg)	Protein (gm)	Iron (mg)	Zinc (mg)	Vitamin C (mg)	Vitamin A (I.U.)	Magnesium (mg)
2 Servings of									
Milk or	1 glass	291	228	8	.1	.9	2	307	33
Cheese	1 oz	204	145	7	.2	.9	0	300	8
High protein foods to provide 20 to 25 grams of protein									
Beef, lean, fat removed	3½ oz	10	191	30	4	6	0	50	21
*Chicken, no skin	3½ oz	13	253	30	1.5	2	0	132	19
*Tuna, canned in oil	3 oz	7	199	24	1.6	1	0	70	24
*Eggs	2	56	180	12	2	1.4	0	520	12
*Baked beans, vegetarian	¾ c	130	231	12	3.8	2	2	113	50
*Lima beans, dried, cooked	¾ c	41	220	12	4.4	1.2	0	0	55
1 serving high Vitamin A and 1 serving high Vitamin C fruit or vegetable									
Orange juice	¾ c	20	30	1	.4	.04	83	370	19
Broccoli	⅔ c	88	62	3	.8	.2	90	2500	24
2 servings other fruits or vegetables and 1 serving potato									
Apple	1	7	10	0	.3	.05	4	90	8
Zucchini	1 cup	50	50	2	.8	.8	20	780	32
Potato, baked	5 oz	13	98	4	1	.5	30	0	33
4 servings of foods from grains and potato (above) or 5 servings of foods from grains									
Cereal, wholewheat, cooked	1 cup	17	127	4	1.2	1.2	0	0	41
Bread, wholewheat	3 sl	72	213	9	2.4	1.5	0	0	66
*Pasta	1 cup	14	85	7	1.4	.7	0	0	36
1 serving poly-unsaturated oil									
Corn oil margarine	1 tbsp	0	0	0	0	0	0	500	0
Total		772	1154	68	11.2	12.1	229	4897	285
RDA, adult female		800	800	46	18	15	45	4000	300
RDA, adult male		800	800	56	10	15	45	5000	350

* Alternate foods not included in totals.

Sodium mg	Potassium mg	Thiamin mg	Riboflavin mg	Niacin mg	Vitamin B-6 mg	Pantothenic Acid mg	Folacin mcg	Vitamin B-12 mcg	Vitamin E mg	Total Fat gm	Poly-unsaturated Fat gm	Cholesterol mg	Carbo-hydrate gm	Energy Calories
120	370	.1	.4	.2	.1	.8	12	.9	.1	8	.3	33	12	150
176	28	+	.1	.02	.02	.1	5	.2	.4	9	.3	30	0	114
60	261	.1	.4	4.5	.4	.5	4	2	1	15	.3	91	0	266
75	377	.1	.1	8.8	.5	1	3	.4	.4	6	1	85	0	182
595	301	+	.1	10	.4	.3	2	2.2	.5	7	.7	50	0	170
292	130	.1	.3	+	.1	1.7	49	1.2	1	12	1.4	504	1	160
647	512	.1	.1	1.1	.2	.3	45	0	.3	1	—	0	45	230
28	872	.2	.1	1.0	.2	.3	183	0	.3	1	—	0	37	197
2	381	.17	.06	.7	.1	.3	102	0	0	0	0	0	19	80
10	267	.09	.20	.8	.2	1.2	56	0	1.9	0	0	0	5	26
1	100	.03	.02	.1	.03	.1	8	0	.6	0	0	0	15	58
2	282	.1	.16	1.6	.1	.3	22	0	2.4	0	0	0	6	28
6	753	.15	.06	2.5	.3	.6	26	0	.2	0	0	0	31	140
5	118	.15	.05	1.5	.1	.2	118	0	.7	0	0	0	23	110
378	216	.27	.09	2.4	.1	.5	48	0	.3	—	0	0	42	195
—	103	.23	.13	1.8	.1	.3	13	0	—	0	0	0	39	190
115	0	0	0	0	0	0	0	0	1.4	11	4	0	0	100
875	2776	1.16	1.54	14.3			401	3.1	9	43	4.7	154	153	1267
		1.00	1.20	13	2		400	3	12					
		1.20	1.50	18	2		400	3	15					

The Backbone of Good Nutrition Foods in Menu Form

BREAKFAST
  1 serving high vitamin C fruit
  1 serving enriched or whole wheat cereal
  1 serving whole wheat bread
  Margarine or butter
  1 cup of whole milk
  (Other foods for calories)

LUNCH
  1 slice whole wheat bread
  Margarine or butter
  Macaroni and cheese
  Vegetable salad
  1 serving fruit
  ½ cup whole milk or yogurt

DINNER
  1 serving meat, fish, or poultry
  Freshly cooked potato
  1 serving high vitamin A vegetable
  Other vegetable or salad
  Margarine or butter
  Mayonnaise or salad dressing
  Dessert and other foods for calories

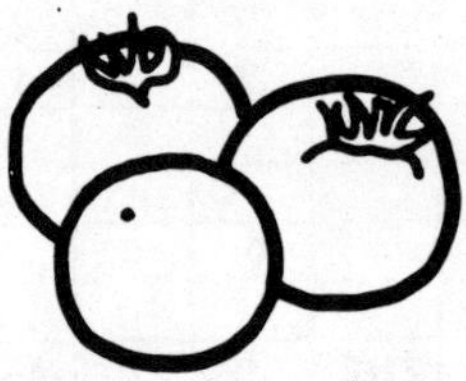

NUTRITIONAL NEEDS OF CHILDREN AND TEENAGERS

Children and teenagers require the same protective or high nutrient density foods as adults for their health, but in increasing amounts as they grow to maturity. Each day they need the following foods. Children under the age of six should not be allowed to fill up on milk, even if they are very fond of it. They require other foods for the other nutrients (especially iron) other minerals and vitamins found in fruits and vegetables. They need all the foods in the basic diet, but in smaller amounts than in the table of essential foods (page 206), which is planned for adult needs. Two glasses of milk will meet their calcium need and with an egg or a very small serving of meat their RDA protein need also. Children require calories for growth and to sustain their great activity as well. Carbohydrate foods such as oatmeal cookies, puddings, bread, and cereals contribute the calories needed, and the B-vitamins required by the increased carbohydrate. Dried fruits, fruit juices, butter or margarine, and peanut butter are also high nutrient sources of calories needed by growing active children.

Between the ages of six and twelve, children need to increase their milk intake, first to three glasses and then to four each day. They may prefer to take some of the milk in the form of cheese. Their intake of all the other essential foods should be increased by giving them larger servings. They also require the other foods suggested above to provide calories for growth.

During the teen years the nutrient and energy needs are the greatest in a man's lifetime. In a woman's lifetime they are equalled only during pregnancy and breast-feeding. Calcium is needed to complete the mineralization of bones. Teenagers who are not very active should perhaps drink skim milk as some of the quart of milk they require daily. They should include the other foods needed for good health. Surveys show that teenagers tend to eat few fruits and vegetables, which results in low vitamin A and trace mineral intakes. Teenagers in this country do not lack protein or calories.

Teenage girls require a constant source of iron. The pregnant teenager has special diet problems. She has the protein and calcium needs of pregnancy before she has completed her own growth of muscle and bone. Teenage pregnancy places both mother and child at risk of nutritional deficiencies. Such girls require special dietary counseling.

	6 to 10 Years	10 to 12 Years	12 to 17 Years
Milk	2 to 3 cups	3 to 4 cups	4 cups (1 qt)
Eggs	1	1	1 or more
Meats, fish, poultry	2 to 3 ounces	3 to 4 ounces	4 ounces
Legumes or Peanut butter	2 servings a week as an alternate to meat 2 tablespoons as an alternative to 1 ounce of meat		
Vitamin C fruit	1 small serving	1 serving	1 or 2 servings
Other fruit	⅓ cup	½ cup	1 cup
Vitamin A vegetable	¼ cup	⅓ cup	½ cup
Other vegetable	¼ cup	⅓ cup	½ cup
Fresh potato	⅓ cup	½ cup	¾ cup
Whole grain cereal	½ cup	¾ cup	1 cup
Whole grain bread	3 slices	3 slices	4 to 6 slices
Butter or margarine	1 tbsp	1 tbsp	1 tbsp

NUTRITION AND ADULTS

When you look at the table of RDA's (page 96) you will see no reduced need for the essential nutrients as you get older, with the exception of vitamin D. It is not certain whether we need vitamin D other than that made in our skin by sunshine after our bone growth is complete. There is, however, a recommended decrease in calories, because of (usual) reduced activity and because there are no longer growth needs.

The college athlete is one person who has to seriously assess his or her food intake pattern on graduating. If he or she gets a desk job and has the usual double cheeseburger and milk shake for lunch and an expense-account dinner he or she can well be starting a pattern of underexercise and over-nutrition that can lead to weight gain and the problems that can arise from it.

Nutrition and the Over-Fifty Group

Again the RDA table makes the suggestion that caloric needs decrease with advancing years. However, if you are well and active you are the best judge of whether or not you are gaining too much weight. If you are well and not overweight you probably have been following good food habits since the 1940's when good nutrition rules were highly publicized. If you have a 5 or even 10 pound margin of extra weight above the weight the tables indicate you may be better able to withstand surgery or some of the illnesses that unfortunately catch up with us.

THE BACKBONE OF GOOD NUTRITION FOR WEIGHT CONTROL

The only healthy way to control your weight is to balance the energy you take in as food with the energy you use up by your activities. The beginning of this chapter outlined the foods you require, in the amounts you require to meet your needs for almost 50 nutrients. The energy in these foods adds up to 1267 calories. So you see you can get all the nutrients you need from foods that contribute several hundred fewer calories than you need. All successful diets for weight loss are based on these essential foods.

Unfortunately a lot of diets for weight loss that have been popularized are based on clinical diets developed for extreme cases of obesity. One example of these diets is the low-carbohydrate, unrestricted fat-and-protein regimen. When you follow such a program you may lose weight, but you have not changed your food habits for the better.

This diet seems to be successful though usually only for a short time. When fat is drawn from your fat cells to be used for energy, at one point in the energy cycle it has to team up with glucose that is also being used, so that the complete fat molecule is oxidized to water and carbon dioxide. The fat is reduced to a substance called a ketone (acetone is a common ketone) at this stage. If there is no glucose being metabolized at the same time the ketones stay, unchanged, in the blood stream. The ketones are acid. Our physiological systems maintain our blood at an amazingly constant composition. When it becomes acid, water is withdrawn from the tissues to correct the blood and so the ketones can be got rid of by your kidneys. Your weight loss is to a large degree water.

A condition of ketosis is not normal and can cause damage to your tissue cells and your bones. A constant state of ketosis can cause a slow withdrawal of calcium from your bones to balance the acid state of your blood. This can lead to the erosion of the bones that hold your teeth, or thinning of other bones, resulting in fractures. There is a similar loss of electrolytes, especially potassium and magnesium, affecting normal muscle function. Potassium is particularly vital for heart rhythm. The phosphorus that is left from the metabolism of protein for energy from a high-protein reduction diet can bring on the same results.

A vegetable plate with a poached egg, or a chef's salad, is a better-balanced low-calorie lunch than the conventional "dieter's special" meat patty with a scoop of cottage cheese in place of the bun. The latter lacks vitamins, minerals, and, most important, fiber.

What You Should Know About Weight-Loss Diets

A weight-loss diet, by its very nature, is a high-fat diet. The fat is from your body stores and it may surprise you to know that it contains both saturated and polyunsaturated fatty acids. If you require 1800 calories a day for your size and activity and take only 1200 calories as food, you are getting 600 calories (66 grams) from your body fat. If you take less food, the proportion of fat calories rises. It is not good for you to draw many more calories from fat unless you are under medical supervision.

You are in no way starving if you are on a reduced food intake. Your desire for food may be starved a bit, but for every 10 pounds you are overweight, you have 35,000 calories in your energy banks to draw on. The concept that your energy supply comes constantly and directly from your digestive tract has been an easy one to obtain from articles in the popular press. We are equipped with a hormonal system that keeps our blood glucose at a quite constant level. After you have eaten, the hormones work to convert the energy from the food into fat and store it. When you are not eating, the system goes in reverse. The fat stores are changed to energy. Your body cells are constantly supplied with energy, quite apart from immediate food intake.

You have probably put on those extra pounds over a long period of time. You may not have changed your eating patterns, but your activities may have decreased. Unfortunately for those who love food, you cannot break the laws of calorie intake and outgo and not gain weight. You cannot eat all you want unless you increase your activities or otherwise do more to use up the energy provided by the foods you enjoy.

Things to Think About if You Are Overweight

- Your excess weight is a self-inflicted load on your physiological system. Only you can decide when and if you wish to change your food or energy-use habits.
- Your body size is determined genetically. If you have large bones, you will always weigh near the top of the weight range for your height as given in the table on page 214. If you have small bones you can weigh the lowest amount. In either case, when you accumulate extra pounds of fat you are putting an extra load of weight on your skeleton to support and carry around. As you get older this can lead to health problems.
- In addition to your body size being determined by genetics so are your heart and vital organs. Your fat cells are not inert tissue but are supplied by blood vessels. Your heart gets an increased load of miles of blood vessels with your increase in body size—a load it was not designed to take. In the same way your genetically sized pancreas can produce only so much insulin. A constant overload for many years can lead to the onset of diabetes when you get older.
- You have trained your system to send out hunger signals by constantly answering with food, especially between meals. Eating snacks does not help you retrain your food habits. Not eating between meals takes the same discipline that is exercised by people who stop smoking. You should not be afraid to feel slight hunger. Remember that at such times you are operating on the energy stored in your fat cells.
- You should never say to yourself that you are "going on a diet" for a certain length of time because you should put out of your mind the idea that when you have lost the weight you wish to lose, you will go back to your former eating pattern. It was obviously a pattern of too much food for your needs. Losing and gaining, and losing and gaining weight has been referred to as a yo-yo pattern. There are indications that such alternating loss and gain has harmful effects.
- You are no different than the average healthy person of proper weight. Everyone has to balance the calories they take in as food and their activity to use them up, to keep at a constant weight. We all have to avoid or eat sparingly the food sources of fat as well as high-sugar and high-fat desserts.

SUGGESTED WEIGHTS FOR HEIGHTS

Height		Median Weight			
		Men		Women	
(in)	(cm)	(lb)	(kg)	(lb)	(kg)
60	152			109 ± 9	49.5 ± 4
62	158			115 ± 9	52.2 ± 4
64	163	133 ± 11	60.5 ± 5	122 ± 10	55.5 ± 5
66	168	142 ± 12	64.5 ± 5	129 ± 10	58.6 ± 5
68	173	151 ± 14	68.6 ± 6	136 ± 10	61.8 ± 5
70	178	159 ± 14	72.3 ± 6	144 ± 11	65.5 ± 5
72	183	167 ± 15	75.9 ± 7	152 ± 12	69.0 ± 5
74	188	175 ± 15	79.5 ± 7		
76	193	182 ± 16	82.7 ± 7		

NOTE: Modified from Table 80 in Hathaway and Ford, 1960, "Heights and Weights of Adults in the U.S.," *Home Economics Research Report No. 10*, ARS, USDA. Weights were based on those of college men and women. Measurements were made without shoes or other clothing. The sign ± refers to the weight range between the 25th and 75th percentile of each height category.

The Way To Healthy Proper Weight

A weight-control diet must supply you with the nutrients you need for good health, but it should not rob you of all the pleasures of dining.

1. It must be deficient *only* in calories.
2. It must have adequate protein but not more than your requirement.
3. It must supply all the minerals and vitamins you need.
4. It must supply adequate fiber for proper functioning of your digestive tract.
5. It should contain just enough fat from food to meet the needs for the essential fatty acid, linoleic acid.
6. You may choose the essential foods you like, but you must be honest with yourself and keep the servings small. Learning to like a wide selection of the high-nutrient foods will give you variety.
7. Your lowered calorie eating pattern should become a way of life.

8. You should eat regular meals and forget snacks.
9. You should expect a gradual, constant weight loss that will be permanent if you have changed your ways.
10. Food habits and food likes can be changed—if they couldn't, none of the new products in the supermarket would have survived.

GOOD NUTRITION WEIGHT-LOSS PLAN

The essential foods with the elimination of 140 calories leaves about 1200 calories of proper nutrition. The 140 calories are easily eliminated by using one glass of skim milk, which is 70 calories less, in place of whole milk, and by using half a serving of potato or omitting one slice of bread, for another 70 calories. At this calorie level, it may be advisable to take a vitamin B supplement that is well balanced and of moderate level. Here is how the 1200 calories can be put in menu form:

BREAKFAST
1 serving high vitamin C fruit
1 serving enriched or whole grain cereal
1 serving whole wheat bread
1 teaspoon liquid corn oil margarine
½ cup skim milk

LUNCH
2 slices whole wheat bread or 1 cup cooked enriched pasta
1 teaspoon of liquid corn oil margarine
1 slice cheese
1 serving vegetable or salad
1 serving fruit
½ cup skim milk

DINNER
Meat, fish, or poultry, 3½ ounces
Half a freshly cooked potato
1 serving high vitamin A vegetable
1 serving other vegetable or salad
1 teaspoon liquid corn oil margarine or salad dressing
1 serving fruit

NOTE: There are several disease conditions in which weight loss is indicated. People with such conditions should not diet on their own but under careful medical guidance. Such therapeutic diets for the overweight diabetic, the extremely overweight person, or people with heart diseases, for example, are beyond the scope of this handbook.

NUTRIENT NEEDS OF PREGNANT WOMEN

Requirements for all nutrients are increased during pregnancy and if you nurse your baby (see the table of Recommended Allowances, Chapter 6). Recent research has shown that the developing baby can be affected by the nutritional deficiencies of the mother. Different nutrients play a role at different times in the development of the unborn baby, so it is essential for the mother to be well nourished throughout her entire pregnancy.

The foods that are the backbone of good nutrition must be the base of the diet. However, in the case of pregnancy, the increased need for calories should be supplied by the same high-nutrient foods as the base diet because all nutrients are needed in increased amounts. It is very important to consume four glasses of milk a day. The mother-to-be should also not gain fat weight, so should eat sparingly of high calorie foods.

How To Feed Your Baby

Research over the past several years has reaffirmed the importance of the proper feeding of infants and small children. The best food for an infant is breast milk. In addition to general health and well-being, the nourishment they receive at periods of rapid growth can affect their whole lives.

An infant must be fed a diet that is adequate in protein, including all the essential amino acids, at the time its brain is undergoing rapid cell growth in order for the brain to reach its maximum genetic development. At another period of rapid cell growth, it is important that the infant not be overfed, since this leads to development of too many fat cells. The number of fat cells we have is a factor in how much fat we can store.

PROPER NUTRITION FOR BABIES*

Hour	Food	1 Month	3 Months	6 Months	10 to 12 Months
6 A.M.	Formula	3–4 oz	5–6 oz	7–8 oz	*Early morning:* ½ piece Zwieback
8 A.M.	Orange juice	1 oz	3 oz	3 oz	3 oz orange juice
	Vitamin D	400 IU	400 IU	400 IU	400 IU
10 A.M.	Formula Cereal	3–4 oz	5–6 oz ¼–2 tbsp	7–8 oz 2–4 tbsp	*Breakfast:* 1 cup milk 2–5 tbsp cereal 1–2 tbsp chopped fruit
2 P.M.	Formula	3–4 oz	5–6 oz	7–8 oz	*Noon:* ¼–1 oz meat or 1 egg
	Egg yolk, hard-cooked Vegetable			1 yolk 2–3 tbsp	2–4 tbsp potato
6 P.M.	Formula	3–4 oz	5–6 oz	7–8 oz	2–4 tbsp chopped vegetable
	Cereal Fruit			2–4 tbsp ¼–2 tbsp	1 cup milk
10 P.M.	Formula	3–4 oz	5–6 oz	Discontinue	*Supper:* 2–5 tbsp cereal or potato
2 A.M.	Formula	3–4 oz	Discontinue		1 cup milk 1–2 tbsp chopped fruit Toast or Zwieback

If the baby is breast fed it is not important to add orange juice and vitamin D as soon.

BALANCING WHAT YOUR FAMILY EATS

In addition to all the engineered foods on the market there has been a marked change in our eating patterns. One of our major nutritional problems today is the lack of balance of the nutritional value of foods eaten by family members who may eat together only occasionally or no more often than once a day. Once upon a time the homemaker had control over the food eaten, or at least had some idea of how well fed the family was. Now many meals are eaten away from home, and this trend will probably continue.

Parents have control over their children's breakfasts when they are small. When children reach school age (and especially if both parents work) parents may have no idea what any member of the family has for breakfast. They have control over their children's lunch when they are small, and if they prepare the lunch the children take to school. If the children have been taught good nutrition they will eat what has been prepared and not trade parts of it with friends. And they will drink the milk supplied. But if they get a prepared lunch, it is difficult for parents to plan a dinner to complete the day's needs, especially if one parent has had a quick carton of yogurt and the other a hearty luncheon.

As eating patterns become more and more individual, and less and less learned from tradition, each of us becomes increasingly responsible for our own health through learning to make good nutritional choices.

Epilogue

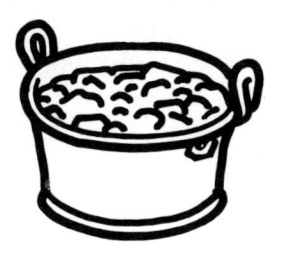

The science of nutrition has been accumulating new knowledge at a rapid pace throughout the 20th century.

This newer knowledge has contributed to better health for millions of people. Nutritional deficiency diseases such as pellagra, scurvy, rickets, beriberi, and protein-calorie malnutrition have been wiped out in some lands and decreased in many. Along with greater medical knowledge and improved health care, nutrition has contributed to lowered maternal and infant mortality and a longer average life span in the United States. Famine and malnutrition still plague many underdeveloped countries. Accelerating population growth threatens world food supply in the years ahead. Food conservation is indicated.

Americans must use nutrition science wisely and recognize what we know and what we do not know. Extensive research is still necessary to unravel mysteries of human nutrition in terms of requirement and balance among all essential nutrients under varying conditions.

Although food technology has been a great boon in preserving food and making it safe from bacteria, we must use technological advances wisely. We must not go beyond our present knowledge of food and nutrition needs in the processing and fabricating and fortifying, of foods.

There are convenience foods as tried and true as dried beans and packaged foods as new as the latest snack tidbit. Some products have failed, and new ones will be tried. As one eminent nutritionist has stated, "The abilities of the food chemist may have outstripped the knowledge of nutrition" in fabricating foods.

Self-control on the part of the food industry can avoid increasing the necessity for government regulation. Curbs on misleading food advertising and marketing techniques can benefit both industry and the public.

Although regulations have been established to inform the consumer of the ingredients of food products, to protect your health, you should base your food intake on naturally occurring foods or on convenient foods that are the true nutritional equivalents.

You, the consumer, must develop greater nutrition know-how in today's more sophisticated food world. At this stage, scientific knowledge should still be tempered with traditional wisdom in the choice of protective, naturally occurring foods.

REFERENCES

Bogert, L. J., G. M. Briggs and D. H. Calloway. *Nutrition and Physical Fitness.* 9th ed. Philadelphia: W. B. Saunders, 1973.

Pennington, Jean. *Dietary Nutrient Guide.* Westport, CN: A.V.I. Publishing.

Taylor, Clara Mae and Orrea Florence Pye. *Foundations of Nutrition.* New York: Macmillan, 1966.

Dietary Goals for the United States, 1977. Washington, D.C.: Superintendent of Documents, U.S. Government Printing Office, 20402.

The Federal Register.

Nutritive Value of American Foods in Common Units. Agriculture Handbook No. 456. Agriculture Research Service, U.S. Department of Agriculture.

Nutritive Value of Foods. Home and Garden Bulletin No. 72. Agriculture Research Service, U.S. Department of Agriculture.

Recommended Dietary Allowances. 8th rev. ed., 1974. Washington, D.C.: National Academy of Sciences.

Index

additives, *see* food additives
alcohol, 171, 177
alpha-tocopherol (vitamin E), 73
amino acids, 10, 16, 40, 134
   chemical nature of, 40, 42, 43
   classification (table), 43
   complementary sources for protein synthesis, 44–45, 137, 160
anemia, 61, 85–86
anti-oxidants, 30, 74, 184
ascorbic acid, *see* vitamin C

B vitamins, *see* vitamin B complex
backbone of good nutrition, 77, 199–205
balance, acid-base, 52, 55, 58
   calcium-phosphorus, 54, 55, 118
   energy, intake and use, 32, 205, 211
barley, 158, 160, 162
beriberi, 13, 77–78
bioflavinoids, 67
biotin, 17, 88
bone problems, 53, 54, 56
bones, building materials for, 51, 105
   how they are made, 51–53
   vitamin needs, 54, 71, 72, 91
botulism, 129
bread, 163–164
breakfast cereals, 163, 165, 167, 170, 197
breakfast pastries, 197
breast milk, 216
butter, 175

calcium and phosphorus, 51–55, 96–97
calories, definition, 22
   diet of 1,200, 215
   food choices and, 200
   protein deficiency, 49
   value of essential foods, 205
   see also energy; food tables
cake mixes, nutritive value of, 194–95

cancer, 129
   Delaney clause regarding, 182
carbohydrates, calories per gram, 22
   digestible, 25
   foods, 22
   glycogen, 26
   how they are made, 23–25
   indigestible (fiber), 23, 25, 27
   information on cereals, 167
   Recommended Dietary Allowance, 27
cereals (grains), 44, 117, 158–60
   breakfast, 165
   nutritive value, 112–13, 168–69
cheese, 110–11
   nutritive value of (table), 112–13
   standards, 114
children, bone problems of, 53
   energy needs of, 209
   foods for, 208–09
   growth, 52
   protein needs of, 48
   RDA, 96–97
   see also infants; teenagers
cholesterol, egg controversy, 134
   role of, in body, 32
chloride, 57
choline, 31, 88
chromium, 65
cobalt, 63, 86
conservation, 119, 219
consumer protection, 107–08, 125, 135, 136, 150–51, 176–77, 181
convenience foods
   additives, 182–87
   future, 219
   ingredients, 188
   nutritional quality, 187–94
copper, 62
corn, 44, 91, 160–61
cream, 175

deoxyribose nucleic acid (DNA), 42
diet, balanced, 198–99
   for children, 209

for infants, 216–17
for pregnant women, 216
for teenagers, 209
for weight loss, 211–15
lacto-ovo vegetarian, 10
vegetarian, 45, 139
diglyceride, definition, 29

eggs, 133–36
energy
  balance, intake and use, 32, 205, 211
  need, basic, 205
  need, constant, 26
  RDAs, 96–97
  sources, 22, 23, 25
  storage, 26–27, 30
  use of fats for, 30
  use of proteins for, 30
enrichment of grain foods, 163, 184
enzymes, definition, 38, 66

fabricated foods, 196–97
fat
  calories per gram, 22
  consumption, 35
  in high protein foods (table), 119
  metabolism for energy, 32
  need for, 33–34
  RDA, 34
  storage, 30–31; *see also* energy
  weight-loss diets high in, 212
fats, chemistry of, 27–29
  cholesterol and, 27–30
  dairy food, 106, 175–76
  digestion of, 31
  food, animal, and plant, 172–73
  food, nutrients in (table), 178–79
  hydrogenated, 29, 174
  of meat, 117
  polyunsaturated, 28, 119, 171
  refined, 173
  saturated, 28, 119, 171
  unsaturated, definition, 28
fatty acids, classification and names, 29
  essential, 33
FDA regulations, 107–08, 129, 152, 163–65, 170, 184–85, 192
fiber, 27, 142, 145, 161, 202
fish, 119, 121, 122–23, 131
fluorine, 64, 185

folacin (folic acid), 68, 84, 85, 96–97, 202
food additives, 182–83
food laws, 98–100, 125, 127, 130, 131, 153, 181, 182; *see also* consumer protection *and* FDA regulations
food rules, 198–99
fortification, definition, 163
  evaluation of, 15
  of foods, 105, 167, 170, 184, 185
freshness dating of meats, 133
frozen foods, storage of, 149–50
fruit drinks, 142, 197
fruits, 82
  canned, standards for, 152–53
  effect of canning on, 147, 153
  effect of freezing on, 148
  nutrients in, 142, 154–55
  storage of, 146–47

glucose, 24–26
glycerol, 27, 31
glycogen, 26–27
goiter, 59–60
grading
  eggs, 135
  meats, 125
  produce, 151
grains, 158
  nutritive value, 159, 168–69
GRAS list, 183

health foods, 89, 93
height/weight table, 214
hesperidin, 67
histidine, 16, 43
hydrogenation of fats, 29, 174
hydrolyzed starch, 159

ice cream, 176
infants
  brain development, 216
  calcium and growth, 52
  energy need, 96–97
  foods for, 217
iodine, 59–61, 96–97, 185
ingredient listing regulations, 188
instant liquid meals, 196
iron, 61–62, 96–97, 201
isoleucine, 16, 43

kwashiorkor, 49

labeling, *see* consumer protection *and* nutrition labeling
lactose intolerance, 107
lacto-ovo vegetarian diet, 10, 136–37, 139
legumes, 122–23, 138–39
linoleic acid, 33, 204
loss of nutrients
  from refining and milling grain, 162, 203
  freezer storage, 149
  cooking, 143–44, 202
leucine, 16, 43
lysine, 16, 43, 44, 160

magnesium, 56–57, 96–97
manganese, 63
margarine, 176
meat
  analogs, 197
  cured, using nitrites, 129
  fat, 117, 119
  grading, 125–26
  how much to eat, 124
  labels, 132
  nutritive value of, 117–23
  perishability of, 127
  protein, 117
  uniform identity naming of, 126
mellorine, 176
methionine, 16, 43–44, 137
milk, 104–07
  forms of, 106, 108–10
  imitation, 196
  intolerance, 107
  nutritional value, 105–07, 112–13, 200
  standards, 107–10
minerals, 16, 51–65
molybdenum, 65
monoglycerides, definition, 29

National Research Council, 94, 164
natural foods, *see* traditional foods
niacin, 68, 81, 82, 96–97
  tryptophan as source of, 82, 120
nickel, 65
nicotinic acid, *see* niacin
nitrates, nitrites in meats, 129
nutrients, essential known, 16–17
  in cake mixes, 193–95
  in cereals, 159

in convenience foods, 187–97
in eggs, 133–34
in fabricated foods, 195–97
in fat foods, 172–73
in fish, 121
in frozen foods, 192
in fruits and vegetables, 142–45
in meat, 117–21
in milk, 105–07
in poultry, 121
in snack foods, 195
nutritional labeling, 98–103, 108, 153
oats, 158, 160–61
overweight, 205, 211–15
osteomalacia, 54
osteoporosis, 54–57
oxalic acid in vegetables, 145

pantothenic acid, 68–84
pellagra, 81, 163
pernicious anemia, 86–87
phenylalanine, 16, 43
phosphorus, 51–55, 118
potassium, 57, 58, 142, 202
potatoes, 149, 161, 156–57
poultry, 121, 131–32
  ingredient listing in products, 131
  Inspection Act, 131
P-P factor, 68
pregnancy, 216
  calcium needs, 53
  iron needs, 62
  protein needs, 48–49
  RDA table, 96–97
protective foods, 12, 199
protein
  allowance, 12
  amino acids, 37
  biological value, 43
  calories per gram of, 22
  chemistry of, 37, 40–43, 137
  deficiency, 49
  energy from, 30, 38, 40
  functions, 38
  in cosmetics, 39–40
  requirements, 46–49, 96–97

ready-to-eat cereals, 165–67
Recommended Dietary Allowances, 27, 34, 94–95, 96–97, 204
rice, 158–160, 164

rice bran extract, 13, 78, 89
rickets, 53–54
riboflavin, 17, 68, 78–81, 96–97, 105
rutin, 67
rye, 158, 160

sausages, 127–29
scurvy, 13, 90
selenium, 65
shortenings, 174
silicon, 65
snack foods, 195
sodium, 18, 57–58, 204
   nitrates and nitrites, 129
soybeans, 139–40
standards, 108–10, 128, 131, 132, 152, 153, 164, 181–82; see also FDA regulations
storage
   cold, 146
   controlled atmosphere, 146
   effect on frozen food, 149
   see also fat
sulphur, 57

teenagers, 53, 62, 199, 208–09
teeth, 51, 53, 64, 167
textured vegetable protein, 124, 140, 197
threonine, 16, 43, 44, 160
thiamin, 17, 66, 68, 76–79, 96–97
tin, 65
traditional foods, 15, 199
triglycerides, chemical equation, 28
tryptophan, 16, 43, 44, 137
   source of niacin, 82, 120

USDA meat inspection, 125

valine, 16, 24
vanadium, 65

vegetarian diets, 10, 45, 137–39
vegetables, 146–49, 152–53
vitamin A, 33, 67–70, 144
   enrichment of milk with, 71, 106, 184
   sources, 69–70, 106, 142, 144
vitamin B complex, 68, 76
vitamin B_1, see thiamin
vitamin B_2, see riboflavin
vitamin B_6, 17, 68, 82–83, 96–97
   sources, 83
vitamin B_{10}, 67
vitamin B_{12}, 17, 31, 86–88, 96–97
   in vegan diets, 139
vitamin B_{15}, 67
vitamin B_{17}, 67
vitamin C, 17, 68, 90
   common cold and, 92
   cooking losses of, 143, 153
   sources, 92, 93, 154–155, 155–56, 202
vitamin D, 68, 71–73, 96–97
   fortification of cereals with, 170
   fortification of milk with, 105, 108
vitamin E, 73–74, 96–97
   sources of, 74, 171, 204
vitamin K, 75
vitamins, list of, 17

water for nutrient transport, 50
weight control, 211–215
wheat, 10, 25, 158, 160–63
whipped toppings, 196

xerophthalmia, 68

yogurt, 110

zinc, 16, 63, 117, 161, 201, 204